PREGNANCY
THE COMPLETE CHILDBIRTH BOOK

PREGNANCY
THE COMPLETE CHILDBIRTH BOOK

NUTAN LAKHANPAL PANDIT

IMPORTANT Please use this book in consultation with your doctor

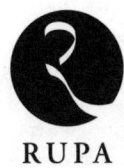

RUPA

Published by
Rupa Publications India Pvt Ltd 2004, 2019
7/16, Ansari Road, Daryaganj
New Delhi 110002

Sales centres:
Allahabad Bengaluru Chennai
Hyderabad Jaipur Kathmandu
Kolkata Mumbai

Copyright © Nutan Lakhanpal Pandit 2004, 2019

The information contained in this book is not intended as a substitute for medical consultation with a physician and may not be construed as medical advice or instruction. Instead, readers should consult appropriate health professionals on any matter relating to their health and well-being. Before starting any diet/exercise, you should speak to your physician. All information contained in this book but not limited to text, graphics, images, information, third party information and/or advice, food, recipes, exercise, diets and psychology are for informational and educational purposes only. No action or inaction should be taken based solely on the contents of this information. This book is not meant to be used, nor should it be used, to diagnose or treat any medical condition. The publisher and the author are in no way liable or responsible with respect to any loss or incidental or consequential damages caused to any person or entity, or alleged to have been caused, directly or indirectly, by use of the information contained in this book.

All rights reserved.

No part of this publication may be reproduced, transmitted, or stored in a retrieval system,
in any form or by any means, electronic, mechanical, photocopying,
recording or otherwise, without the prior permission of the publisher.

ISBN: 978-81-291-0454-0

Eighth impression 2019

10 9 8

The moral right of the author has been asserted.

Printed by Replika Press Pvt. Ltd, India

This book is sold subject to the condition that it shall not, by way
of trade or otherwise, be lent, resold, hired out, or otherwise circulated,
without the publisher's prior consent, in any form of binding
or cover other than that in which it is published.

*This book is dedicated to
my sons, Pranav and Akshaya*

*Also to my aunt, Pushpa Sharma,
whose encouragement and blessings have led me
to take Natural Childbirth Classes*

CONTENTS

Acknowledgements ix
Pregnancy Beliefs xi

1. BIRTH WITHOUT FEAR — 1
Pain Perception — 1
The Brain, the Boss — 2
Sympathetic Nervous System — 2
Muscle Action — 3
The Body's Design for Birth — 3
Experiences of Women — 4

2. YOUR ANATOMY — 6
The Development of the Baby — 8

3. PREGNANCY — 10
Blood/Urine Test — 10
Planning a Healthy Baby — 11
Genetics — 12
Pre-Conception Care — 12
Antenatal Visits — 13
Blood Tests During Pregnancy — 13
Urine Test — 16
Internal Vaginal Examination — 16
Abdominal Examination — 17
Ultrasound — 17
Ultrasound and Safety — 18
Non-Stress Test (NST) — 18
Amniocentesis — 19
Anti-Tetanus Injection — 19
Medical Termination of Pregnancy — 19
Boy or Girl? — 20

4. COMMON PROBLEMS IN PREGNANCY — 22
Physical Changes — 22
Behavioural Changes — 28
Digestive Problems — 31
Urinary Tract Infection — 33
Conditions Needing Special Attention — 35
Toxaemia and Pre-Eclampsia — 36

5. DIET IN PREGNANCY AND AFTER — 40
Eating for Two — 40
A Parasite — 40
Foods You Need — 40
Genetically Modified Crops — 42
Wholesome Foods — 44
Tea, Coffee and Cola Drinks and Chocolates — 46
To Avoid Putting On Too Much Weight — 46
Body Weight — 47
Diet in Labour — 48
Diet when Breastfeeding — 49
Our Traditional Recipes — 50
Ghee — 51
Tips on Weight Control — 51

6. SOME SIMPLE EXERCISES — 54
Neck Exercise — 54
Shoulder Rotation — 55
Deep Breathing — 55
Bust Exercise — 55
Pelvic Floor Exercise — 56
Ankle Movements — 57
Forward Backward — 58
Pelvic Lift — 58
Knee-Chest Position — 58
Leg Lift — 59
Curling Leaf — 59
Leg Swing — 60
Pelvic Tilting — 60
Walking for Cramps and Arches of the Foot — 61
Squatting — 61
Aum Breathing — 62
Relaxation — 62
A Prayer — 64

7. SEX DURING PREGNANCY — 65
Bleeding — 66
Intercourse — 66
Breast Stimulation — 67
After the Birth — 67

8. LABOUR TIME — 68
Fluid Leak — 69
Positions to Adopt in Labour — 70
Upright Position for Labour — 71
Backache in Labour — 72
When on the Drip — 72
Comforters — 73
For a Backache — 74

9. BREATHING AND RELAXATION FOR LABOUR — 76
Ignorance-Fear-Tension-Pain Syndrome — 76
Quick Relaxation in Labour — 76
Breathing for Labour — 77
Conditioned Reflex — 77
Breathing Patterns — 78
Concentration Breathing — 80
Concentration Breathing Can be Used as Distraction Breathing — 80
Not-Pushing Breathing — 81
Transition Breathing — 81
Pushing Breathing — 82

10. INDUCED LABOUR — 84
The Estimated Date of Delivery — 84
Planned Caesarean — 85
Different Methods of Induction — 86
Home Induction — 88
Prolonged Pregnancy — 89

11. BIRTH — 92
Prepared Childbirth — 94
The Baby at Birth — 96

12. VAGINAL BIRTH AFTER A CEASAREAN SECTION (VBAC) — 97
The Caesarean Scar or Incision — 98
Signs of Scar Rupture — 99
When There is a Rupture — 100
Layered Healing of the Uterine Scar — 100

13. DO I HAVE A CHOICE? — 101

14. GENTLE BIRTH — 109

15. BREASTFEEDING — 113
Why should I Breastfeed? — 113
Does Breastfeeding Make Breasts Sag? — 114
How does the Baby Feed? — 114
How to Feed — 115
Colostrum — 115
Fat-Rich Hind Milk — 116
Breast Size — 116
Feeding Bras — 117
Bra Size — 118
Wearing Your Bra — 118
Flat Nipples — 119
Breastfeeding at Birth — 119
Rooming-in — 120
Exclusive Breastfeeding — 120
Constant Feeding Demand — 121
Let Down Reflex — 121
Leaking Breasts — 121
Feeding When Ill — 122
Medication — 122
To Stop Feeding Suddenly — 122
Breast Preparation for Feeding — 122
When Feeding — 123
Forerunner to Milk — 124
Colostrum — 124
Second Night Syndrome & Skin to Skin — 124
Absence of Skin to Skin — 126
Mature Milk — 126
Engorgement — 126
How to Deal with Engorgement — 126
To Express Breast Milk — 127
Breast Pumps — 127
Storing Breast Milk — 128
How to Feed Expressed Breast Milk — 129
If The Baby's Nose Gets Blocked — 129
Feeding Time — 130
Relax When You Feed — 131
Night Feed — 131
Foremilk and Hind Milk — 132
How to Tell If the Baby is Hungry — 132
Will my Milk be Enough? — 133
Less Milk — 133
Burping the Baby — 134
How to Position the Baby — 134
Position after Caesarean Birth — 135
Twins — 136
How to Position Twins — 136
Bonding — 136
Contraceptive effects of Breastfeeding — 137
Breast or Bottle — 137
How Long Should One Feed Last? — 138
How Long to Breastfeed? — 138
Breastfeeding and the Working Woman — 139
The Bottle and Nipple Confusion — 140
Milk Powder — 140
Cow's Milk — 141
How to Sterilize Bottles — 141
How to Bottle-feed — 142
Problems During Breastfeeding — 143
Thrush/Candida Infection — 144
Blocked Ducts — 145
How to Deal with a Blocked Duct — 145
Mastitis (Inflammation of the Breast) — 146
Prevention of Mastitis — 146
Babies With Problems — 147
Cleft Palate — 150
How to Feed a Baby by Cup — 150

16. AFTER CHILDBIRTH — 152
After a Normal Birth — 152
A Sling for the Baby — 154
Exercises After a Normal Delivery — 154
After a Caesarean Section — 155
Post-natal Depression — 158

17. CONTRACEPTION — 160

18. CONDITIONS THAT MAY REQUIRE SURGERY AT BIRTH BY DR MEERA LUTHRA — 168

19. TERATOGENESIS BY DR ASHA SINGH — 170

RECOMMENDED READING — 173

INDEX — 176

ACKNOWLEDGEMENTS

I would like to thank Mrs. Merry Wood, the lady from Canada, who taught me breathing practices before my first delivery; the staff of the National Childbirth Trust, London, for permitting me to attend study days, workshops and childbirth classes when I went to London; Dr Michel Odent, who allowed me to watch how he conducted squatting deliveries, and for showing me his unit replete with facilities for water birth and an operation theatre; Dr S.K. Bhandari for her encouragement.

I am grateful to Dr R.L. Bijlani for his invaluable help with my manuscript.

Thanks to the following persons for helping me with the completion of my book: Dr Asha Singh, Dr Meera Luthra, Dr Kanwal Hazuria, Dr Nalini Singh, Dr Kamla Tiwari, physiotherapist Daulat Dastoor, Dr Jayant Banerjee, Dr Prakash Punjabi, Dr Ratna Zafar Hussein, Dr Ashima Abbott, Dr Preeti Bijlani, Malka Punj, Ashwini Mehta, Sangeeta Gupta, Nita Seth, R. Maniraj, Nirupam Chatterjee, Chitra Sharma and Pradeep Kapoor.

Nutan Lakhanpal Pandit

For classes in natural childbirth, contact:

Nutan Lakhanpal Pandit
Natural Childbirth Centre, D-178, Defence Colony, New Delhi 110 024
Tel: 24601689, 24629951, 9910210409
email: nutanpandit@yahoo.com
website: http://www.ncbchildbirth.com
Facebook: Nutan Pandit Lamaze Program Community

Ideally contact for classes in the 5th month of pregnancy
so that you can attend the course in the 6th month.

PREGNANCY BELIEFS

MYTH: The pain is unbearable.

FALSE! In case of unbearable pain, nature's safety mechanism makes one pass out, i.e. lose consciousness. In labour, women are rendered unconscious by drugs but never by pain. The right attitude to contractions can make it pretty easy to bear. There have been women who have experienced pain-free labour without epidurals/drugs.

MYTH: Have a spoon of ghee daily to lubricate your nerves.

FALSE! To make yourself supple, you need exercise, not ghee. Ghee will make you fat. Be active so that your joints are not rusty and creaky. Earlier, women would work in fields, milk cows, churn butter or grind wheat, hence they could digest the ghee.
However, a little bit of ghee in the diet is essential (see pp. 50–51).

MYTH: The umbilical cord is attached to the mother's navel.

FALSE! The umbilical cord is attached to an organ inside the womb called the placenta. (The placenta is also called the afterbirth since it is delivered after the baby.) This organ prepares and passes the food and nutrition to the baby, through the umbilical cord, which at the other end is attached to the baby's navel.

MYTH: Be happy, read good books.

TRUE! If you are afraid or under stress, the chemistry in your body changes as stress hormones are released. The baby living within, senses the tension the mother is going through. It is therefore important for the mother to strive to be happy.

MYTH: Push when in labour.

FALSE! If you begin to push in early labour before you feel the natural urge to push, there is a possibility of the baby's head, hitting against an unopened cervix (mouth of womb). As a result the baby's head and the cervix become swollen/tender/painful.

MYTH: Walk when in labour.

TRUE! The best thing you can do is to walk when in labour. Gravity hastens the baby's descent, and therefore shortens labour. Also, when you lie on your back, the weight of your baby and uterus press on a major blood vessel called the vena cava, hence reducing the supply of blood to you and your baby. Further, less pain is felt when a woman walks in labour (See box on p. 70 for when to not walk in labour).

MYTH: Eat for two.

FALSE! One does not need to eat for two people, but it is important to eat fresh, nourishing and homemade food during pregnancy. (A working woman can make extra portions and freeze some portions for use when there is not enough time to cook.) The baby grows in such a way that it takes all that it needs, whether the mother has enough or not. For example, a lack of calcium in the mother's diet will cause the calcium from the mother's bones to go to the baby. If a mother does not eat well, she will deplete her health.

MYTH: If you sit cross-legged on the floor, it flattens the baby's head.

FALSE! The best thing you can do is to sit cross-legged, this will exercise the pelvic joints, the very joints that 'open up' when the baby is being born.
With regular exercise, the joints become flexible and open easily at birth. Mopping the floor in the traditional way (using bucket/water/mop) also exercises these joints.
The baby is safely ensconced in the womb and gets no direct pressure on his head when the mother sits cross legged on the floor.

MYTH: Baby gets suffocated if you pull in the stomach.

FALSE! The baby does not suffocate, since it gets oxygen through the umbilical cord, which is attached to its navel and to the placenta at the other end. If you pull in your stomach, the weight of the baby is borne by the pelvic bones and your stomach muscles get a respite from constant stretching. This reduces overstretching of these muscles and minimizes low back pain.

MYTH: Have a glass of milk and ghee or have badam milk before going to hospital.

FALSE! If you have started labour and feel like eating something, eat something light. Once labour has established, if you have something heavy like badam, ghee, milk, you'll feel like vomiting (see pp. 48–49).

MYTH: Bind abdomen after delivery.

FALSE! If you make a jumble of your clothes and fling them in the cupboard, they'll fall on your face when you open it next. If you push your muscles back with a girdle, they'll flop out again. It is important instead to do mild exercises for the first forty days or three months and more vigorous ones later to build back tone in your muscles (see pp. 154 & 155). Binding the abdomen may help to keep the joints in place and prevent post-birth pain in this area which happens if these joints do not go back to their original position. However, care should be taken not to bind so tightly that the abdominal bulge migrates to below the chest and/or it blocks circulation, making the mother uncomfortable.

MYTH: If the cord is around the neck it is going to be a Caesarean section.

FALSE! Babies are often born with the cord wrapped loosely around their necks. The delivery can be normal.

MYTH: If the baby is in breech presentation, that is, feet first, it will be a Caesarean section.

FALSE! If the baby is breech early in pregnancy, it is likely to turn to a head-down position a few weeks before the estimated date of delivery. If it does not turn to a head-down position in a woman having her first delivery, doctors tend to perform a caesarean birth. Experienced doctors and midwives can deliver breech presentation babies normally.

One month before the estimated date of delivery, homoeopathic medicine taken from a classical* homoeopath could turn around a breech baby. Also, stimulation of an acupressure point B67 at the base of the nail of the little toe is known to turn around a breech baby.

MYTH: The baby comes on the expected date of delivery.

FALSE! Labour starts on estimated date of delivery in only 4% of cases.
One week on either side in 50%, 2 weeks earlier and 1 week later in 80%, at 42 weeks in 10% and at 43 weeks plus in 4% of cases.

Source: Textbook of Obstetrics by Dr D.C. Dutta

---

*A classical homoeopath is one who asks innumerable questions about how you feel mentally, what illnesses your parents had, what your likes and dislikes are, etc.

BIRTH WITHOUT FEAR

One truth we gain from living through the years, Fear brings more pain than does the pain it fears.

JOHN GOLDEN

CHILDBIRTH IS A natural and universal phenomenon, and yet the knowledge of it among average women is rather haphazard, incomplete, or distorted.

A woman generally has a vague notion that childbirth involves unbearable pain and danger. This notion is formed as a result of the distorted tales heard during adolescence or later. What can be pieced together from gossip, movies or fiction draws a picture of passive pain, to which a woman has to submit in utter helplessness. A negative attitude during labour causes her entire body to tense up with fear.

If one undergoes unendurable pain, one passes out as a rule, i.e. loses consciousness. This is nature's safety mechanism. However, women in labour may be rendered unconscious by drugs, but never by pain. Hence, what pain can be felt, can be endured.

PAIN PERCEPTION

Pain and childbirth have been associated with each other for so long that normal uterine contractions are often referred to as pain.

Uterine contractions and pain have become synonyms. A woman is often told that pain is the signal of labour. In France, labour wards in many units are referred to as the 'Hall of Pain'. Women who have had babies also talk of 'the pain' hence a temporary connection between words and nerve centres takes place.

The uterine nerves signal the beginning of labour to the brain. The brain translates it inevitably into pain, anticipating it.

When the human body is healthy and functioning efficiently, the organs constantly send streams of messages to the brain to inform it of their working. Coming from various internal and external sources, these messages have to compete with each other. Hence many of them get ignored completely.

However, when the potential force of the brain is reduced, say, by shock, we can painfully feel the working of internal organs, e.g. shocking news can cause a stomachache or a pain in the throat.

In labour, the potential force of the brain can be reduced by a whole lot of negative feedback over a period of time, resulting from the expectation of unbearable pain. In other words, if you expect pain, it can impair the normal activity of the brain, and make you feel greater pain. Each negative feedback regarding labour received over the years has the same effect as drops of

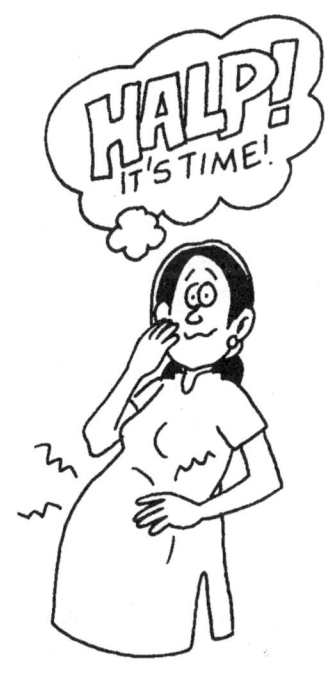

water falling regularly at the same spot on a hard stone. Millions of drops do succeed in making a dent.

It is therefore important to think positively about labour. Think of it as a natural experience. As you grow up you experience menstruation, intercourse, and then childbirth. It is a normal and natural function of your body. When labour is allowed to be natural and drug-free the body releases endorphin hormones that are natural painkillers and give a feeling of well-being.

THE BRAIN, THE BOSS

When a woman is in labour, the uterus contracts. Stimulus is received and sent to the brain by the nerve endings in the uterus. If the brain interprets it as 'fearful pain' the protective mechanism which advocates flight or fight will take over a woman's body. As a result, the woman, incapable of flight, will fight each contraction by building up muscular tension throughout her body. Along with general muscular rigidity, her uterus will also become rigid and offer resistance to the uterine muscles working towards birth. This is perceived as pain.

However, if the woman understands that the strain her body is undergoing is part of the physical strain associated with the expulsive efforts of her uterus, of which she has no reason to be afraid, the contractions will be a new experience for her. The muscles of her uterus will work unhampered by fearful tension and with each contraction get closer to birth, so that the woman will have a shorter, less painful, labour.

Hence the pain a woman will feel in labour will greatly depend on her brain's interpretation of 'pain', as either something fearful or as something to work with.

SYMPATHETIC NERVOUS SYSTEM

When the sympathetic nervous system is stimulated by fear, it restricts the blood flow to and from the uterus. In the absence of adequate fuel and no effective means of disposing of waste products, no organ can function optimally. This is one of the most serious influences of fear on the reproductive organs, and is directly responsible for many of the unpredictable complications of an otherwise normal labour.

According to Langley and Anderson (1893-94), stimulation of the sympathetic nerves to the uterus by fear causes the uterus to appear pallid, firm and bloodless, but when the stimulation is removed, it rapidly fills with blood and becomes an elastic, deep pink uterus. A bloodless, white uterus can lead to urgent distress of the fetus and a Caesarean may have to be performed.

Impairment of circulation is a cause of pain, because the blood flow is too weak to dispose of the byproducts of metabolism. Restricted circulation can also give rise to severe pain in the muscle tissues of the uterus thereby prolonging the process. Even if the bodily organs are in order, e.g. the pelvis is adequate for the baby's head, and the baby is in the correct position for coming out, psychological fear and its associated pain—not real pain—can make labour long.

Fear and its effects not only prolong labour but are also responsible for haemorrhage and tissue injury in the mother, and anoxaemia (less than normal concentration of oxygen in the blood), respiratory failure, and exhaustion in the newborn.

MUSCLE ACTION

All over the body there are sets of muscles that work in harmony with each other. For example, the muscles in front of and behind the upper arm. Try raising your arm and feel the muscles in front of your upper arm tense. Then lower your arm and feel the muscles in the back of your upper arm tense. Now tense both these muscles together and feel the arm becoming rigid. If the contraction is strong and maintained for some time, the whole arm will quiver and in a short while, there will be considerable pain in the arm.

The same kind of harmonious muscle action is seen in the uterus during childbirth. The uterus is made up of many muscle fibres. One set of muscle fibres is longitudinal, that is, they run from the mouth of the womb, over the front, top and back of the uterus. Contraction of these muscle fibres brings about the expulsion of the baby from the womb. Then there are circular fibres concentrated in the lower part of the uterus, near its mouth or outlet. The stretching and relaxing of these fibres opens the mouth of the womb. However, if the circular fibres stiffen, they will cause the cervix or mouth of the womb to close and hold up or inhibit the activity of the uterus. This uncalled-for rigidity caused by tense muscles can make labour longer and more painful. (see pg. 76)

THE BODY'S DESIGN FOR BIRTH

A woman's body is designed for giving birth. To begin with, a woman's pelvic bones are broader than a man's. A woman's pelvis is heart-shaped, whereas a male pelvis is apple-shaped.

After the baby has passed through the cervix or mouth of the uterus, it makes its way through the vagina. The vagina is made up of folds and is therefore capable of unfolding, just as the pleats in front of a saree can unfold. As the baby passes through the vagina, it opens up to make way for the baby. The more relaxed the muscles of the vaginal passage, the less tension the baby's head encounters during birth.

The cranial or head bones of the baby are not fused. As the baby's head negotiates the birth canal, these bones can mould to the size of the vaginal passage. They can also override each other if necessary. At birth the bones come back to their original shape. It is because of this that some babies are

THE FEMALE PELVIS

There are three joints in the female pelvis that spread apart at birth. Two are at the back, on either side of the sacrum i.e. the lower portion of the backbone where it joins the iliac bones or the basin-like bones of the pelvis. These are called the two sacro-iliac joints. Then there is one joint in front of the pelvis, called the symphysis pubis. These three joints spread apart to make way for the baby's exit.

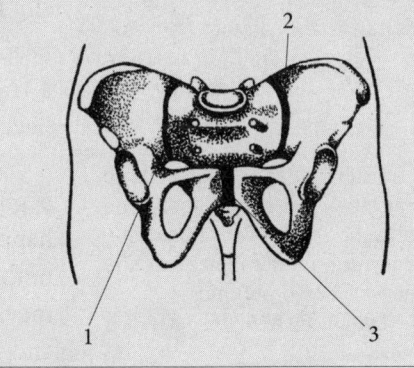

> One must have positive feelings—that's what counts. You can face anything.
>
> NEHA BALI
> Computer based training developer
>
> I tried to help her by reminding her and helping her to concentrate and breathe.
>
> VIVEK BALI
> Neha's husband
>
> Found that the breathing and relaxation helped tremendously. Thanks to the classes and exercises, I did not feel at all apprehensive and on the whole found labour not difficult to bear.
>
> RUKSHANA SHROFF
>
> Labour was absolutely wonderful. I knew exactly what to expect—the breathing was great—otherwise my mom had said she would not be able to see me through the labour pains. Breathing helped me so much that it was almost painless.
>
> AMRITA KHOSLA
> second delivery (first by Caesarean)
>
> Like a Buddha she would sit up and mumble something each time a contraction came—I thought she was muttering her mantra but she said it was her breathing.
>
> VANDANA JAGWANI'S MOTHER

---

born with funny bumps on their heads, which smooth out in a few days.

The body releases hormones to control the process of birth and make it pain-free.

An interesting fact is that uterine contractions and their associated 'pain' form a very short part of the total labour. For instance, if you have 1-minute contractions every 5 minutes, it will mean that in 1 hour you will have 12 minutes of contractions and 48 minutes without them. At the start, contractions could be every 15 minutes and last for 30 seconds. So in 1 hour, one would have only 2 minutes of contractions.

EXPERIENCES OF WOMEN

More than 4,000 women have gone through childbirth preparation classes conducted by the author. Many have felt more confident about the birth experience, and have gone through it with little or no pain.

A psychologically prepared woman can handle any kind of labour confidently. Says Rita, who had a Caesarean section: 'Around 4.30 a.m. there was a heavy flow of blood as the placenta had started separating from the uterine wall. It was accidental haemorrhage. By the time I was operated two-thirds of the placenta had separated and there was foetal distress. The best thing about my delivery was my cute baby girl whose life and mine were saved by timely treatment administered to me by my efficient doctor, as my case had become very serious.'

When a woman understands that in her case a Caesarean section is necessary, she accepts the decision consciously. Moreover, since she has been handling her labour with breathing and relaxation, she is in good mental and physical health. Since she is calm and collected, she will let the anesthetist send her to sleep with a greatly reduced amount of anesthesia, so that both she and her baby will experience less discomfort afterwards. At the same time, when women become knowledgeable, they will not accept anything blindly.

When a woman has not prepared herself at all for giving birth, and she fears it, she may be filled with a dread of labour. Each contraction will become a signal of pain and therefore pain will result. On the other hand, a trained woman can have a very positive attitude towards birth and may have a smooth and easy labour.

There is one category of women who fail to make progress once labour begins. Throughout pregnancy they display no anxiety and appear to be happy. But once labour begins, they lose heart, and begin complaining that nothing is happening and often end up with slow progress, long labour, and maybe a Caesarean. Such a woman is one who suppresses her innate fears and leaves them buried in her subconscious mind, only for them to surface at the time of labour, hampering the normal sequence of events.

In Dr Dick Read's book, Childbirth Without Fear, a case is mentioned that illustrates this point. There was a physiotherapist who had been 'a very keen exponent of relaxation and preparation for childbirth'. She had a very easy and trouble-free first labour, with minimum discomfort. When she had her second baby, she suddenly experienced very strong contractions. They were so strong that she immediately suspected that something was wrong. She suddenly lost her nerve and literally began to 'scream the place down.' She was immediately given inhalation analgesia and brought under control, and the baby was born normally. She later admitted that she had expected her second labour to be easier than her first, and when she had felt more discomfort than expected, she had thought the worst and lost control of herself, so that fear took over. In the labour following her second one, she had a comparatively easy time again, since the circumstances of her fear had been explained to her. She understood that no two labours are alike, and that sometimes in second and subsequent labours strong contractions are experienced.

Fears repressed into the background can lead to problems during birth. So it is important for every pregnant woman to come out with her fears or imaginings, to discuss them, and understand them. No two labours are alike; each labour is different. Even in one woman, two labours will not be alike. Divest yourself of any preconceived notions about labour. There is no right or wrong, perfect or imperfect in labour. Your labour just happens, you cannot set specific goals for it.

You simply equip yourself with some knowledge, relaxation and breathing techniques. This will help you to cope with labour by using simple, non-pharmacological methods like moving about to find a comfortable position when the discomfort of a contraction happens.

Natural childbirth implies having one's baby the natural way, that is, with a relaxed attitude, without anesthesia or analgesics and without any mechanical aid to birth.

NATURAL CHILDBIRTH

An interesting description of a woman in labour is given in Dr Dick Read's book *Childbirth Without Fear*, London, 1977, which influenced Dr Read to such an extent that he became a pioneer of natural birth in Britain.

He describes the incident thus: 'In due course the baby was born. There was no fuss or noise. Everything seemed to have been carried out according to an ordered plan. There was only one slight dissension: I tried to persuade my patient to let me put the mask over her face and give her some chloroform when the head appeared and dilation of the passage was obvious. She, however, resented the suggestion and firmly but kindly refused to take this help. It was the first time in my short experience that I had ever been refused when offering chloroform. I asked her why she would not use the mask. She looked from the old woman who had been assisting, to the window through which was bursting the first light of dawn and then shyly turned to me and said: "It didn't hurt. It wasn't meant to, was it, doctor?" I began to realise that there was no law in nature and no design that could justify the pain of childbirth.'

2 YOUR ANATOMY

IT IS IMPORTANT for every woman to understand the anatomy of her body. To do so a woman should freely feel and examine her body. Do not be shy of your body. Most women are not aware of the appearance of their sexual organs as compared to the other parts of their body. Women tend to consider themselves unclean 'down there' and have as little to do with the area as possible.

It is good to know that the vagina, which has a natural self-cleansing process, is cleaner than the inside of the mouth. Feel good about your body, it is not unclean or obscene. It is you. Get familiar with yourself. You are unique in your ability to reproduce. Each month your periods reaffirm your fertility. Take a mirror and have a look at yourself 'down there'. Lie down on the bed, bend legs at knees. Place feet flat on the bed, move thighs apart and hold a mirror between them. In a mature woman the single most obvious feature will be the pubic hair.

If you look lower down from the pubis, which is the fatty hair-covered mass just below the lower abdomen, you will notice your sexual as well as your excretory organs. You will notice an area shaped like the alphabet A, within the outer hairy flaps. The two arms of the 'A' are the lips of the vagina. The tip of the A, which is on top, has in it the clitoris and the hood of the clitoris, which is the most sensitive spot in the area. The clitoris becomes erect during sexual arousal, just as the penis becomes erect during sexual arousal in a man. Within the lips of the vagina, and below the clitoris, there are two openings or orifices. The small opening just below the clitoris is the urethra from where urine is passed. Below the urethra is a larger opening, the vagina. Your vagina is the opening through which the menstrual flow passes, and through which your baby will be born. It is made up of folds which afford it elasticity. These unfold when the vagina expands during intercourse or childbirth. Below the vagina, further back, is the anus. Through the anus stool is passed. The urethra leads up to the bladder, a bag in which urine collects before urination. The anus leads up to the rectum, the last part of the large intestine where faecal matter collects before being expelled as stool.

The uterus is the organ that is going to carry your baby when you

1. Pubic hair
2. Clitoris
3. Urinary Opening
4. Vaginal Opening
5. Anus
6. Perineum

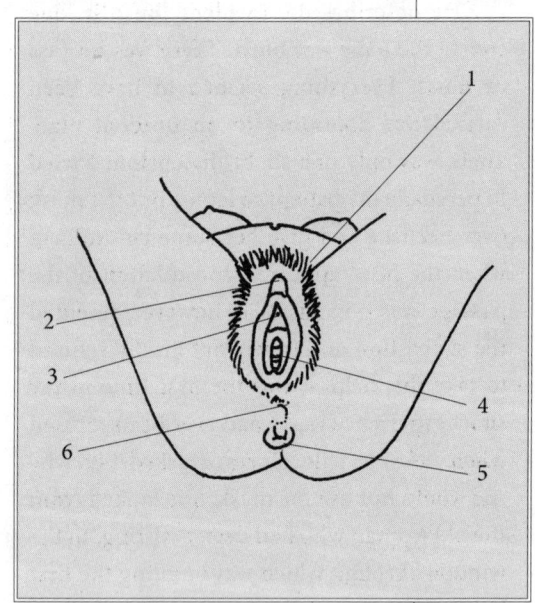

get pregnant. It has thick walls and lies between the bladder and the rectum. It may be folded backwards or forwards slightly, in which case it is called retroverted or anteverted, respectively. This corrects itself in pregnancy and will not cause complications at birth. Its upper part is called its body, and the lower, narrower part is called the cervix or mouth of the womb.

If you wash your hands and insert a finger in your vagina, you can touch your cervix since it protrudes into the vagina. It feels like a dimpled nose tip or like a chin. The entrance into the uterus through the cervix is very small and is called the os.

The top part of the uterus has two openings on either side that lead to a fine tube on either side, called fallopian tubes. The other end of the tube is funnel-shaped and leads to the ovaries on either side. The ovaries are two in number and the size of an unshelled almond. They are placed on either side of the uterus. The ovaries have 2 functions. They produce the female sex hormones—oestrogen and progesterone. They also produce the ovum or egg which is wafted into the fallopian tube on being released. It is then fertilised by the sperm, which travels from the vagina, through the cervix, into the uterus, and from the uterus to the fallopian tube.

The fertilised egg then journeys back to the uterus from the fallopian tube and houses itself in the body of the uterus, where it begins to grow. As the fertilised egg grows, the thick walls of the uterus thin out as it enlarges and balloons up with the pregnancy. In rare instances the fertilised ovum implants itself not on the wall of the uterus, but in the fallopian tube, and very rarely in the abdominal cavity, on the ovary or the cervix. Such a pregnancy is called an ectopic pregnancy and surgery is normally required to end it.

The sign of an ectopic pregnancy is sharp abdominal pain. Pain due to ectopic pregnancy is aggravated by body motion, such as bending over, rising or travelling in a car. Discomfort connected with ectopic pregnancy usually occurs in the first 3 months of pregnancy.

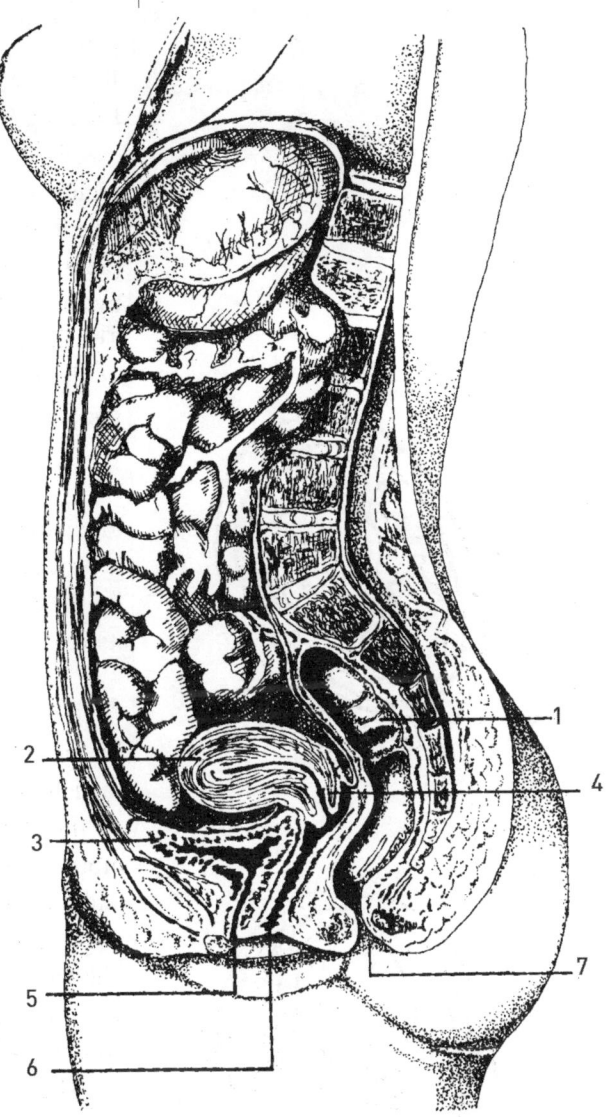

1. Rectum
2. Uterus
3. Bladder
4. Cervix
5. Urinary Opening
6. Vaginal Opening
7. Anus

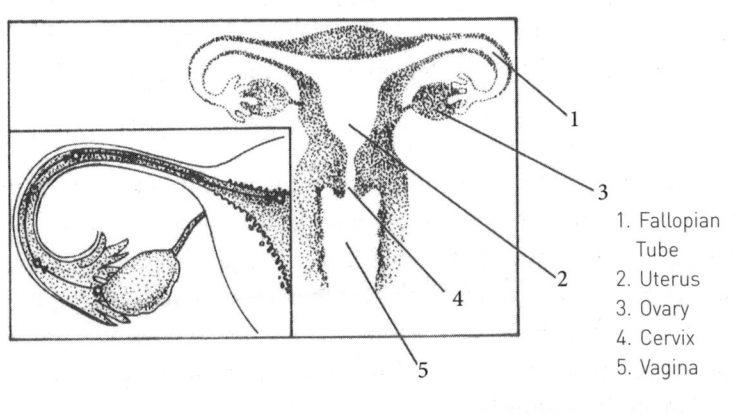

1. Fallopian Tube
2. Uterus
3. Ovary
4. Cervix
5. Vagina

THE DEVELOPMENT OF THE BABY

It can be divided into three specific periods of 3 months each, together totalling 9 months.

By the end of the first 3 months the baby is about 3½ inches long. The vital organs and limbs are fully formed but not sufficiently developed. The amniotic sac contains about 3.5 ounces of amniotic fluid and the fetus has plenty of room to move about, although the movements will not yet be felt by the mother. The heart is beating, the eyes, though closed, are in position. The facial features are properly formed and the ears are in place on the sides of the head. The sex organs are developed so that the baby has a male or female identity.

THE FIRST TRIMESTER: 1-3 MONTHS

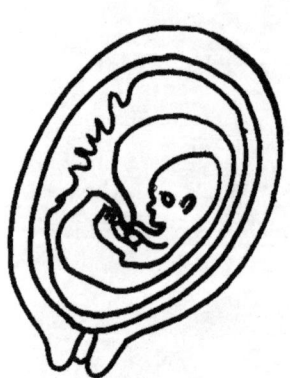

The fetus swallows the amniotic fluid, most of which is used by its body, and it produces drops of sterile urine. The amniotic fluid is constantly refreshed by the amniotic sac. As the baby is not breathing, it does not choke. It gets its oxygen from the mother's bloodstream through the umbilical cord.

THE SECOND TRIMESTER: 4-6 MONTHS

By the end of the second trimester the baby is about 14 inches long, roughly the length of his mother's fist and forearm, and weighs about 1 kilogramme. At the start of the second trimester, or from the 4th month onwards, the mother begins to feel movements of the fetus, and she begins 'to show'. The fetus can now smile and suck its thumb. At the ends of the fingers and toes, ridges develop, giving the baby a unique identity of fingerprints.
The trunk and legs of the fetus lengthen and the head no longer looks too large for the rest of its body. Eyelashes and eyebrows appear, although the eyes remain closed until the end of this trimester.

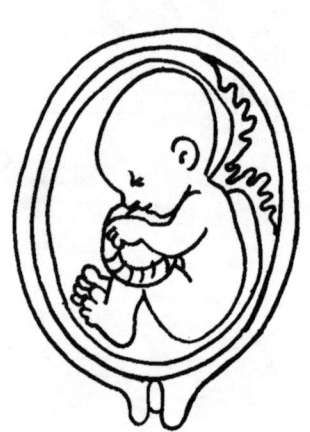

The skin begins to grow a coat of fine, downy hair called lanugo, which is shed before or shortly after birth. During this period the baby also develops a whitish greasy coating called vernix from the oil secreted from its skin and dead skin cells.

The fetus now swallows a pint of amniotic fluid daily and returns it to the amniotic sac through urination. The amniotic fluid is recycled every hour, when one-third of it is absorbed into the mother's bloodstream and replaced with fresh fluid secreted from the amniotic sac.

THE THIRD TRIMESTER: 7-9 MONTHS

During the last 3 months the baby gains weight, and slowly grows to reach right up to the mother's breastbone. As the fetus becomes large it can no longer move freely as before, since it gets cramped for space. So now instead of movements of the fetus, the mother feels its kicks and pokes.

During this trimester the baby stores protein to build muscles, calcium for its bones, iron for its red blood cells, fat to insulate it against changes in temperature after birth.

By the end of the 7th month the fetus' brain matures to be able to cope with breathing and swallowing. Thumb sucking is now resorted to more frequently. If born at this stage the baby has a 90% chance of surviving.

By the end of the 8th month the fetus looks quite like what it will at birth. Although the lungs are not yet fully operational, the baby has a 95% chance of surviving if born at this stage.

It is during the last trimester that the fetus' eyes open. The senses undergo their greatest development at this stage. The hair on the head grows and fingernails and toenails develop.

Sometime during the 9th month the fetus generally turns head-down in the womb. About 2 weeks before birth, it descends about 2 inches, settling in the mother's pelvic bones. This is called lightening, engagement, fixing, or dropping of the head.

The mother feels lighter as the pressure of the fetus pushing on her diaphragm and lungs is reduced, and she can breathe more easily. Mild contractions of the muscles of the womb may be felt in the 9th month as the womb turns the baby into the head-down position or as the womb prepares its muscles for delivery. Sometimes babies are born feet first. Such babies are called breech babies.

1. Uterus/Womb
A muscular organ in which the baby lives until birth.

2. Placenta/Afterbirth
A tissue growth on the inside of the uterus. It is delivered after the birth of the baby, after its need and function are over; hence the name afterbirth. The placenta matures towards the end of pregnancy.

3. Umbilical Cord
A rope of blood vessels attached to the baby at its navel on one end and to the placenta on the other. Through it nutrients reach the baby.

4. Amniotic Sac/Bag of Water
A membrane sac filled with liquid called amniotic fluid, in which the baby floats, and which acts as a shock absorber, protecting the baby in case of accidental knocks.

5. Cervix
The mouth of the uterus, leading to the birth canal. The baby passes through the muscular opening at the cervix and then through the birth canal to the outside world.

6. Mucus Plug
A plug of mucus and blood, that plugs the cervix much as a cork plugs a bottle. It prevents infection from entering the womb.

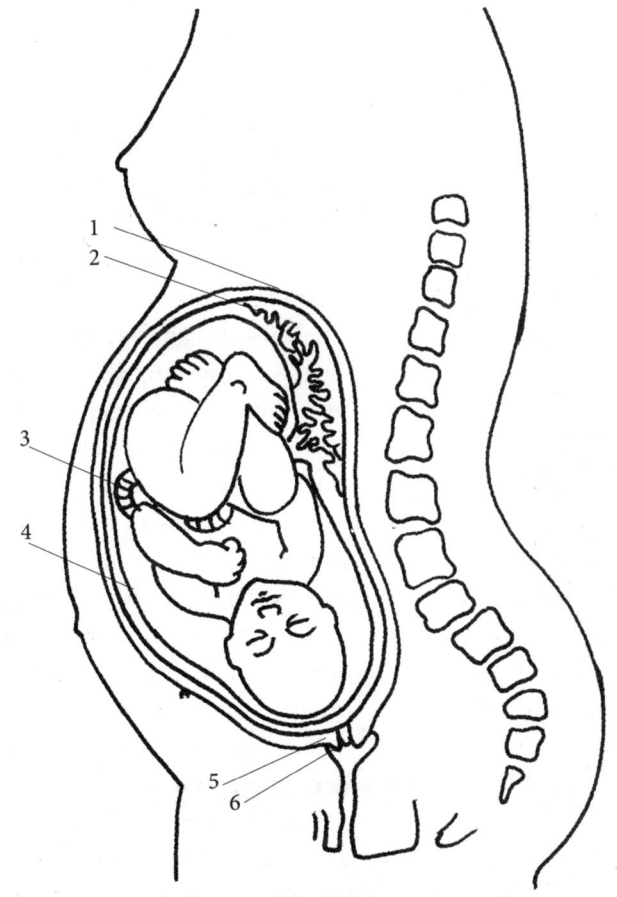

3 PREGNANCY

THE SIMPLEST WAY of knowing that you are pregnant is the missed period. Along with a missed period a woman may feel nauseous, may need to urinate more frequently and feel tenderness in the breasts. When you go to the doctor in order to reconfirm your pregnancy the doctor will check you for an enlarged uterus, softening of genital organs and during an internal vaginal examination the cervix will be seen to have taken on a purplish-velvety look, typical of pregnancy.

BLOOD/URINE TEST

A blood or urine test can help detect the presence of a pregnancy. The blood or urine is tested for the presence of HCG, human chorionic gonadotropin. The developing placenta begins to produce this hormone to prevent menstruation and protect the pregnancy. For an earlier result the blood test is more reliable. High-dose hormone tablets used to be given earlier to test pregnancy. It would make the period occur if there was no pregnancy. If there was a pregnancy and if the fetus was female there was a possibility that the tablet could produce masculinisation. Tablets are not used to test for pregnancy anymore. Instead, tablets with a different hormonal combination are now used to abort an unwanted pregnancy. If tests or a visit to the doctor confirm that you are pregnant, you must immediately start taking care of yourself and your baby by eating nutritious food, avoiding too much tea, coffee, and colas, stopping alcohol, tobacco, and indiscriminate use of medicines and tranquilisers.

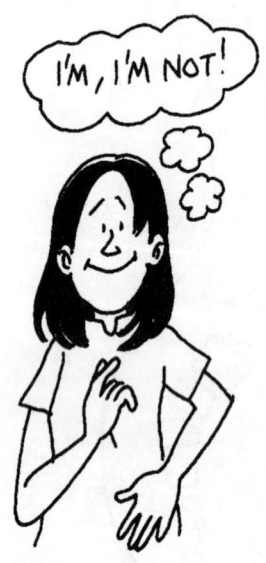

When you visit your dentist or general physician tell him that you are pregnant, because medicines of all kinds should be avoided, particularly in the first 3 months of pregnancy. The thalidomide tragedy in 1962 jolted people into realising that drugs taken by the mother affect not only her but also the baby. Thalidomide was a sedative prescribed to women in early pregnancy. Over 5,000 children throughout the world were born with limb defects, in some cases with no limbs at all. Drugs that affect the rapidly developing fetus in the first 12 weeks are called teratogenic.

As Dr Gordon Bourne says in *Pregnancy*, 'Teratogenic drugs should not be given at any stage of pregnancy. These include thalidomide, phenytoin, anti-thyroid drugs, anti-cancer agents, some sex hormones, alcohol, tetracycline and some anesthetic agents.' Only a doctor will be able to judge the correct dose of a drug, should it need to be used. If you are a patient of diabetes or epilepsy you must not stop your medication without consulting your doctor. Any medicine should be taken strictly under the doctor's supervision, even if it is only an aspirin.

Many ancient cultures like the Indian, Japanese and Chinese stress that the mood and activities of a pregnant woman should be positive and happy, since they believe that what the mother is exposed to in pregnancy affects the growing baby within her. Hippocrates tells of his belief that a pregnant woman directly influences the baby she carries.

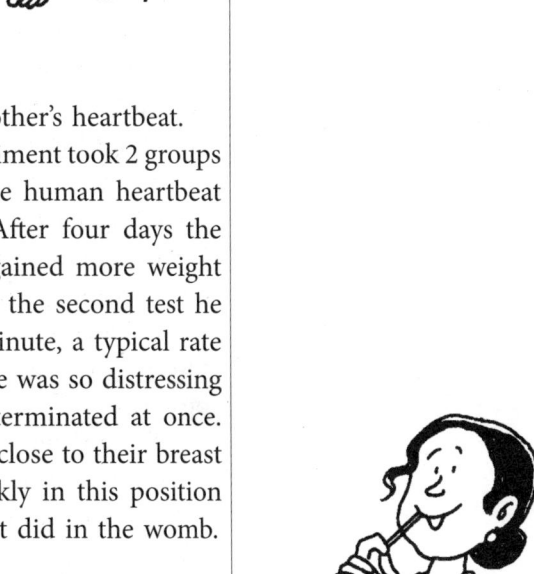

According to a legend, when Confucius' mother became pregnant, she withdrew to a mountain to pray and gave birth to Confucius there. In ancient China a pregnant woman was told not to look at ugly things, not to listen to rude talk, not to speak about trivial matters and not to listen to gossip.

Take time off to relax (see p. 62). Researchers have recently inserted small microphones into the uterus and recorded what the fetus hears. The womb, they find, is full of the mother's bodily music; the whooshing bowels, the gurgling stomach and the mother's heartbeat.

Dr Lee Salk, a leading psychologist, in his classic experiment took 2 groups of infants. One group was exposed to a recording of the human heartbeat of 80 per minute. The second group was unexposed. After four days the group exposed to the sound of the beating heart had gained more weight on an average, as compared to the unexposed group. In the second test he played a recording of a heart beating at 120 beats per minute, a typical rate achieved in an anxious or frightened adult. The rapid rate was so distressing to the newborn babies that the experiment had to be terminated at once. Little wonder that mothers the world over hold the baby close to their breast to comfort it. It could be that the baby is soothed quickly in this position because it hears the familiar pulsation of the heart that it did in the womb.

PLANNING A HEALTHY BABY

Today, with means of contraception easily available and the number of working women on the increase, a pregnancy is often planned and not accidental. If you are a diabetic, your condition will need to be assessed before your pregnancy to avoid complications later.

To conceive, all contraception should be stopped. If you are on the pill, you should go off it, and switch to the condom and spermicidal pessaries for 2 to 3 months, so that all hormones are out of your system by the time you conceive. Biologically it is best to have your baby in your 20s. Risks increase in the under-20s and over-40s, and slightly in the over-30s.

GENETICS

Each of us carries two copies of genes. One from the father, and one from the mother. If both copies of the genes are abnormal then a person can get disease.

With the help of technology it can be assessed whether the normal gene has been passed to the child, or the abnormal gene. This was not available till the 1980s.

Earlier, to find a problem DNA sequence had to be done and its cost was lakhs of rupees. Now a new technology has been developed called Next Gen Sequencing. Blood is taken and checked for genes. It costs 25,000 to 30,000 rupees.

Internationally research is underway to make this test as simple as possible.

When people marry their cousins, it increases the chances of the bad genes coming together. Hence, in consanguineous marriages the new generation has a greater chance of abnormality.

Certain abnormalities like Down's Syndrome can be detected by ultrasound. However, some abnormalities like thalassaemia or muscular dystrophy can be detected only by these special tests.

If a disease is detected, it can be treated by the exon skipping technique, so that the disease is less severe. In this technique the cellular machinery is encouraged to skip one exon.

Earlier it was believed that genetic diseases are not treatable but now, according to Dr I.C. Verma, Centre of Medical Genetics, Ganga Ram Hospital, Delhi, even in common diseases like diabetes, hypertension, genetic solutions are available by determining genetic compositions.

In India consanguineous marriages are the most common cause of genetic diseases. It is therefore important to not marry a cousin if there is a genetic problem.

There is now a new branch of medicine called epigenetics. It refers to the external modifications to DNA that turns genes on or off. Epigenetics is the reason why a skin cell looks different from a brain cell. Both these cells contain the same DNA, but the genes are expressed differently (turned on or off), which creates the different cell type. Epigenetics literally means above genetics.

PRE-CONCEPTION CARE

A few months before you plan to conceive, have a blood test taken to check if you are anaemic. If you get your anaemia under control, it will go a long way towards producing a healthy baby. So eat foods rich in iron (see p. 40). Eating wisely is important both for you and your husband. A nutritious diet, less stress, less alcohol and cigarettes, less lead exhaust from vehicles, less caffeine from tea, coffee and cola drinks, no indiscriminate use of drugs, are all factors that will contribute to a strong and healthy baby. If you and your husband can check these factors before you conceive, it should give a strong foundation to your baby. You should check these factors 3 to 6 months before conception, especially approximately 15 days before the next period is expected, because the pregnancy starts at that time. Always check these factors throughout pregnancy. A man's diet, smoking and drinking habits, etc., can harm his sperm. It is being increasingly proved that health and nutritional status of both the man and the woman before conception are very important.

A couple who takes care of all these factors have done their best to produce a healthy baby. It may require a slight alteration of lifestyle, but it will give you a healthier baby and mother. A healthier mother will be able to cope more easily with the care of the baby later.

During pregnancy keep up your normal activities but do not overwork. Avoid lifting heavy things, as it can lead to a miscarriage. Regular exercise will help you keep fit (see p. 54). Normal activities will help keep your muscles toned, making your delivery easy.

ANTENATAL VISITS

When you become pregnant, you must consult an obstetrician or an obstetrics OPD in a hospital or a medical centre. Often, 3 months may pass by the time a woman goes for consultation. Under medical guidance you will go through pregnancy and birth with fewer complications. Any potentially dangerous situation will be controlled through preventive measures. For instance, a woman with a rhesus-negative blood group will be given an anti-D immunoglobulin injection after the birth of her first baby so that her second delivery will be problem-free. A rhesus-negative woman, who has not had an anti-D injection after her first delivery or after an abortion preceding her first delivery, may have a baby that will need a complete blood transfusion at birth (see p. 37).

A woman with swollen feet, hands and face will also need to follow simple medical advice so that other complications do not crop up. Blood pressure and weight will also be checked during antenatal visits.

The doctor will ask about your previous pregnancies, miscarriages, abortions, about when you had your last period, what contraception you have been using, what illnesses you have suffered from, etc.

Until the 7th month you will be called for a check-up once a month. Until the 9th month you will be called every 15 days and then every week until you go into labour. The doctor will prescribe certain tests.

BLOOD TESTS DURING PREGNANCY

A blood test will be taken to find out the haemoglobin content of the blood. Haemoglobin is the red colouring matter of the blood that carries life-giving oxygen to all parts of the mother's body, including the baby. Haemoglobin levels tend to fall in pregnancy and could drop to as low as 9.5 gms/100 ml (see p. 37).

Using knees and legs for lifting heavy things

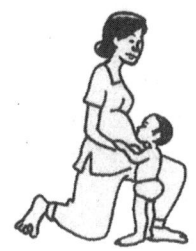

Step 1
Standing close to a child or object, put one foot forward and drop to one knee.

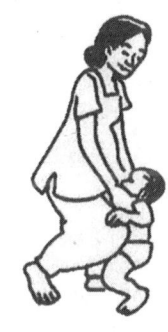

Step 2
Rise to your feet keeping your back straight and lifting with the front leg while the back foot balances.

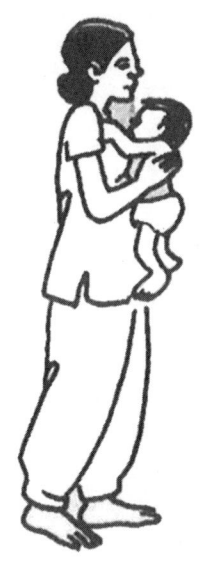

Your blood group will also be noted, in case you need a blood transfusion in an emergency. The blood will be checked to see if it is rhesus-negative or rhesus-positive (see p. 37). A blood test, Hbs Ag, is also recommended sometimes to test for hepatitis.

VDRL-VENEREAL DISEASE RESEARCH LAB TEST

The Venereal Disease Research Lab test is a blood test that checks for the presence of any sexually transmitted disease or venereal disease. If, for instance, a woman is found to have syphilis, she can give birth to a deformed child. Both the woman and her husband should have the VDRL test. Even if it turns out that one of them has the disease, both will receive a course of antibiotic injections to protect themselves and the baby. It is important that both partners cooperate with the doctor.

There may be other instances when the doctor would prescribe a blood test. Medical supervision is therefore essential.

AFP-ALPHA-FETO-PROTEIN TEST

The Alpha-Feto-Protein test is a specialised blood test that can reveal if there are any major defects in the baby. The mother's blood is checked for alpha-feto-protein which is a protein that is produced by the baby's liver and is passed to the mother's bloodstream through the placenta. It is most accurate between 16 and 18 weeks of pregnancy. If the test suggests that the baby is not normal, it should be repeated. If the second test gives similar results the fetus also should be checked by an ultrasound scan and amniocentesis.

TRIPLE MARKER TEST

The triple marker test consists of three tests, conducted through a blood sample from the mother:

1. The AFP test as mentioned above.
2. The HCG test, tests for the presence of the hormone 'human chorionic gonadotrophin', a hormone produced by the placenta.
3. The Estriol test, tests the presence of an estrogen hormone which is produced by both the fetus and the placenta.

This is a screening test. It does not diagnose a problem, it only suggests whether further testing is required or not. It is more likely to be recommended if a problem is suspected in the pregnancy, regarding the well-being of the baby. It can also help date the pregnancy if there is confusion about the dates. If it indicates there may be a problem, the test is repeated. The second test often clears the fear of something being wrong.

The result of this test is known to be inaccurate. It therefore often creates unnecessary stress for the mother and family.

DOUBLE MARKER TEST

The double marker test is performed from the 9th to the 13th and half weeks of pregnancy, after performing an ultrasound scan.

The ultrasound scan measures the thickness on the back of the baby's neck (called the nuchal fold). A thickness higher than 3.5 is not good.

The double marker test is a blood test that checks for two things:

1. HCG or human chorionic gonadotrophin hormone. A high or low level of this hormone would indicate if the baby has Down's Syndrome or a chromosomal defect called trisomy, which means the presence of three sets of chromosomes instead of the usual two.
2. PAPP or pregnancy associated plasma protein. A low level of this protein would also indicate Down's Syndrome or trisomy.

A positive result indicates a high risk; a negative result indicates a low risk.

TORCH

A comprehensive blood test called TORCH tests the blood for various infections like toxoplasma, syphilis, rubella or german measles, cytomegalovirus, and herpes or Hepatitis B.

When these infections are found present they may manifest in the child in the months following birth. If they are already present then their treatment can begin at birth. For instance, immunisation against Hepatitis B can be given to the baby in the weeks following birth if the infection is present in the mother. Likewise, treatment for toxoplasma or syphilis infection can be started at birth. In other words, prior knowledge of any infection can make it possible for early diagnosis and appropriate medical care for the child.

PETS, GARDENING, RAW MEAT (TOXOPLASMA)

Toxoplasmosis is a parasitic infection that can be acquired from soil, cat faeces and raw meat.

It is an infection present in birds and animals. It is also a common dormant infection in humans. Its presence in humans varies from population to population, but it is more prevalent in warmer, more humid climates.

A woman who has already been infected by it before becoming pregnant will be immune to it. Her baby will not be threatened by it. It is only when a woman acquires this infection in her pregnancy that the baby could be affected by it. Approximately 50% of women who acquire this infection and are not treated can pass it to the baby. However, if this infection is identified and treated with antibodies (spiramycin, for instance) it reduces the risk of damage by 50% to 60%. Infection can result mainly in abnormalities of the brain and growth retardation.

The damage caused by this infection is greatest in mothers who acquire this infection in the first three months of pregnancy. (Interestingly, the incidence of transmission of infection to the baby is least in early pregnancy, and greatest in late pregnancy.)

To prevent this infection a woman can follow simple guidelines. She should eat only well-cooked meat and eggs, and drink only pasteurised milk or boiled milk. Avoid handling raw meat. If handling raw meat, the hands should be washed immediately, and kitchen surfaces and vessels washed well thereafter. Do not touch mouth or eyes while handling raw meat. Wash fruits and vegetables before consumption. Protect food from flies and cockroaches. When gardening or handling faeces of animals use gloves.

HIV/AIDS

A blood test checks for the Human Immunodeficiency Virus. A person who tests positive for HIV has a strong possibility of developing AIDS (Acquired Immuno-Deficiency Syndrome), in which case the person's immunity or strength to fight infection falls drastically so that the person picks up all kinds of infections like cold, respiratory and skin infections, etc. If a woman is suffering from AIDS she can pass the infection to her newborn baby.

The time of transmission of infection to the baby could be within the womb or at the time of birth. Breast milk can also transmit the infection. A child born to an HIV-infected mother should have regular investigative tests until the age of 6 to 8 months to check if the child has got the infection from the mother or not. If the mother has HIV infection, pregnancy can increase her chance of developing AIDS.

However, if a woman is known to be HIV or AIDS infected and gets pregnant, recent research has shown that the use of two standard drugs, AZT and 3TC, can block the passing of the virus from the mother to the baby. Recent research also shows that without treatment 17% of babies can be infected, whereas with treatment the infection of babies can be lowered to 11% if the two drugs are given when labour begins, and continued for a week after birth. The medicine can be given to the mother when labour starts and it must be given to both mother and child for a week following birth. This is to protect the child from exposure to HIV-contaminated blood and secretions as well as from virus in the breast milk, which causes 1/3rd of all infections in the young.

The risk of infection can be further reduced to 9% if treatment is begun 26 weeks before delivery and continued for a week afterwards.

A new drug, nevirapine, is also known to reduce the transmission of HIV from mother to baby, and costs much less than AZT. Nevirapine is administered to an HIV-infected woman in labour, and another dose is given to the baby within 3 days of birth.

URINE TEST

A urine test is routine in pregnancy. The urine will be analysed for infection, and for glucose which will show up if there is diabetes. Ketones may show up if you are vomiting a lot or not eating enough. In late pregnancy albumin or protein in the urine will indicate pre-eclampsia (see p. 36).

INTERNAL VAGINAL EXAMINATION

An internal examination could be done at the start of pregnancy and at its end, and sometimes during its course. At the start of pregnancy it could be done to confirm the pregnancy and exclude any possibility of abnormalities of the pelvis, vagina, or cervix.

At the end of pregnancy it could be done to check the readiness of the cervix or its ripeness. It does not harm the baby. It will help if you breathe out slowly through the mouth while it is being carried out, and relax your pelvic floor as you do when passing urine.

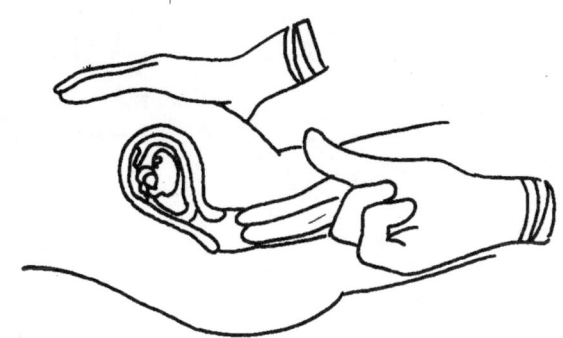

ABDOMINAL EXAMINATION

When you go for a check-up the size and shape of your abdomen will be felt by the doctor after making you lie down. The doctor will examine your abdomen for its shape and size, for abdominal scars and for the movements of the fetus. By palpating your abdomen with one or both hands the doctor can gain a lot of information about the size of the baby, in what position the baby is lying, and the presentation of its head.

The height of the growing uterus also gives an idea of the growth of the baby. At 3 months the uterus can be felt in the lower abdomen, rising out of the pelvis. At 5½ the uterus reaches the height of the navel. At 7½ months the uterus will be halfway between the navel and the breastbone, or the region below the breasts. In the 9th month the uterus will reach the area below the breasts.

ULTRASOUND

Ultrasound was first used during the Second World War to detect submarines. In a pregnant woman, sound waves are directed to the fetus inside the uterus, and as they bounce off the baby's bones and tissues, a picture of the fetus appears on a TV screen. The picture may not make much sense to you, but the expert working the machine will be able to interpret it. It is really quite simple. Even a novice would be able to differentiate the dark areas, which are fluid-filled, from the white areas which are solid.

When you go for an ultrasound scan, you must have a full bladder. You will be made to lie down next to the machine and an oily substance will be spread over your abdomen. A small flat device will be moved slowly all over your abdomen during the scan.

It is a fairly new technology that began to be widely used in obstetrics in India only from the early 1980s. In other words, it is in its infancy. It does not appear to harm the mother or the baby in any way but there is no evidence that it is completely safe either. It took 40 years to discover the harmful effects of the X-ray, which was the only technique of getting some information of the baby in the uterus before the ultrasound scan.

As a diagnostic tool the ultrasound is invaluable, since it can give the doctor vital information on diagnosis of pregnancy, missed abortion, hydatidiform mole, ectopic pregnancies, twin pregnancies, the position of the fetus and placenta, the age of the fetus, abnormalities of the fetus or uterus. Scans should be done in pregnancy if the doctor thinks it advisable for investigative purposes. As a routine procedure it is avoidable.

It is not necessary that you must have a routine ultrasound scan during every antenatal visit.

According to *Mayes' Midwifery* (1997), 'An ultrasound scan is usually performed between 16 and 18 weeks gestation'; an ultrasound done between 16 and 20 weeks gives an accurate idea of how old the pregnancy is. All other information about the baby is also sourced most accurately at this time. After 24 weeks, the baby's age in the uterus cannot be accurately predicted by an ultrasound.

An ultrasound done approximately between 16 and 20 weeks is often referred to as 'Level Two Ultrasound'. Its results are most accurate. If at all you are to have an ultrasound during your pregnancy this could be the one, since it is done after the baby's organs and body are fully developed.

ULTRASOUND AND SAFETY

According to Marjorie Tew, in her book, *Safer Childbirth?* (1995), 'It has never been tested whether there is an upper safer limit to the number of scans, though now there is some evidence that birth weight is lower after several scans. Nor is it known whether safety is related to a scan's duration, which can vary widely in length, or to the power of the instrument used, which also varies widely between models, newer models usually being much more powerful than the older ones used in the 1970s. 'Studies which showed that the ultrasound was safe were done when women were given only one ultrasound scan, in the sixteenth week; after all the vital organs had been formed.'

TRANS-VAGINAL ULTRASOUND

Exposure to the baby can be greater with the vaginal ultrasound as it bypasses the protection of the mother's body.

NON-STRESS TEST (NST)

This is not a test for all pregnant women. If required this test is likely to be done in the last three months of pregnancy i.e. in the 7th, 8th or 9th month. It is done as a precaution to test the well-being of the baby.
Mostly, this test is used if the pregnant mother is going past her due date. It may also be done on mothers in the ninth month of pregnancy if they have diabetes, high blood pressure, low amniotic fluid or any other medical problem that may require monitoring the well-being of the baby in the womb.

The mother is made to lie down and a device is strapped onto her stomach. She may be asked to press a button when the baby moves so that the heart rate can be seen in accordance with the movement. If the baby is not moving the mother may be asked to eat or drink something. Or, the technician may try to wake a sleeping baby with a loud sound. The test can take about 30 minutes or more.

The result of the test may be reactive (normal) or non-reactive (not normal).

If the result of the test is reactive, it means that your baby is doing fine. Sometimes doctors like to repeat the test again after a week or so.
If the result is non-reactive it doesn't necessarily mean that there is something wrong with the baby, it only means that the result has not provided enough information and you may have to take the test again in an hour or so, or the doctor may advise some other tests. However, a non-reactive test could also indicate that the baby is not doing well in the womb and the doctor may decide to induce labour.

AMNIOCENTESIS

This is a procedure where a small amount of fluid is taken out from the pregnant mother's abdomen (amniotic sac) to test for chromosomal and other abnormalities. It is not a routine test. Under local anesthesia a needle is inserted into the mother's abdomen and a little bit of amniotic fluid is withdrawn. This is done along with an ultrasound, so that the placenta and the fetus are not disturbed by the needle. The fluid, which contains fetal cells, can then be analysed for the detection of abnormalities of the nervous system, mental handicaps, including Mongolism or Down's Syndrome, inherited disorders, etc.

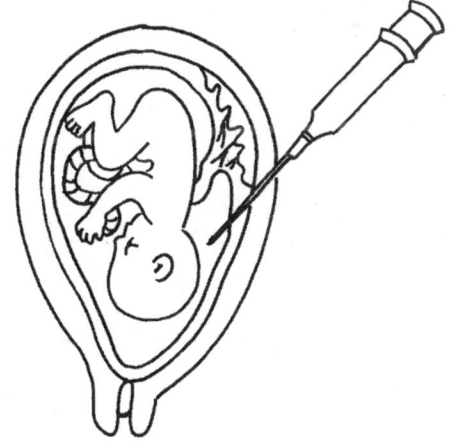

Even though it might be carried out efficiently under hygienic conditions, there is a 1-2% chance that it might lead to a spontaneous abortion. Besides, the couple should first decide what they want to do with the results of the test. If the tests suggest an abnormality, are they ready to opt for termination of the pregnancy? This can be difficult, for the test cannot be done before 14 weeks of pregnancy, when a termination would mean having an induced labour. If a woman already has one abnormal child, she might want to consider this test. She should seek the advice of her doctor.

ANTI-TETANUS INJECTION

Anti-tetanus injections are given routinely to all pregnant women. An anti-tetanus injection taken by the mother in pregnancy protects both the mother and the baby from tetanus infection for up to several months after the birth. It is usually given in 2 doses, in the 26th week and 6 weeks later.

MEDICAL TERMINATION OF PREGNANCY

Amniocentesis or the AFP test may suggest the baby has a severe abnormality of the spine or brain. If you catch an infection of German measles or rubella in the first 3 months of pregnancy it can physically and mentally handicap the child. Chickenpox can do similar things. In such cases the doctor would advise an abortion. It is better to go for an abortion than to live with an abnormal child for the rest of your life with a guilty feeling that you could have avoided all this pain to yourself and your baby. Discuss things with your doctor and if you like, with a psychotherapist as well.

Medical termination of pregnancy is now easily available and quite safe. It is offered by public hospitals and private clinics. It should not be resorted to as a contraceptive method, in which case repeated abortions can seriously harm a woman's health.

BOY OR GIRL?

When the ovum is fertilized by the sperm, 23 chromosomes each are contributed by the male and the female, making a total of 46 chromosomes. Of the sex chromosomes, one is contributed by the male and the other by the female. These are the famous XX (girl) chromosome present in the female and the XY (boy) chromosome present in the male. The mother always contributes the X chromosome. The sex of the child is determined by the father's contribution of the sex chromosome. If it is X the baby born will be female. If it is Y the baby born will be male.

There are some not very scientific theories that claim to be able to tilt the balance towards the conception of a male or female child, as desired. One such theory propounded by a French doctor, Francois Papa, claims that if a woman follows a particular kind of diet for 2 to 3 months before conception, she can choose a male or female baby.

Some doctors in Canada and France have been advocating the diet theory and say it has an 80% chance of success. For a girl, they advise a diet rich in starch, milk and milk products, and low in salt. They also recommend taking a tablet of calcium every day. For a boy, they advise eating a high salt diet, with plenty of meat and fruit. Milk and milk products are not permitted. A daily potassium tablet may also be recommended.

According to *The Complete Handbook of Pregnancy* edited by W. Rose-Neil, research studies have shown that the more often you have intercourse, the more likely you are to have a boy. More boys tend to be born, for example, in the first few years after marriage, immediately following a reunion after a long parting, and in younger parents.

The timing of intercourse is also said to influence the sex of the child. If conception takes place within 48 hours after ovulation you are more likely to have a male child. Within 48 hours of ovulation, intercourse should take place at least 3 times, and then one should refrain until the next period. The opposite would apply to conceive a female child. That is, intercourse should take place 48 hours after ovulation to conceive a female child. In order to pinpoint the exact time of ovulation, ultrasound clinics offer a package deal. You are called for an ultrasound every day, 3 days after your period is over. You have to go early in the morning on a full bladder. You go until the ultrasound detects that ovulation has taken place.

Another way to pinpoint ovulation would be the temperature method (see p. 161).

Douching is also said to influence the sex of the child. An alkaline vaginal douche before intercourse is said to help conceive a boy. An alkaline vaginal douche can be made of 1 tablespoon bicarbonate of soda dissolved in 500 ml of warm distilled water. To conceive a girl, an acid douche can be made from 1 tablespoon of white vinegar and 1 tablespoon of warm distilled water. If you are very keen on conceiving either a daughter or a son you could try these methods or discuss them with your doctor.

4
COMMON PROBLEMS IN PREGNANCY

MOST OF THE common ailments during pregnancy are minor and can be relieved by simple changes in lifestyle. As a result of tremendous changes occurring in the body, discomfort, muscle pulls, bleeding gums and cramps are some of the accepted problems a pregnant woman is likely to encounter. However, some lucky women never face any problems at all. Consult your doctor if you are in doubt about your symptoms.

PHYSICAL CHANGES

DARKENING PIGMENTATION

With pregnancy it is common to develop a darkening of certain areas of the body, like the darkening of the nipple and areola; or the darkening of a line starting from below the navel and ending at the pubic hair; or the development of dark patches on the face.

These are caused by pregnancy hormones. These hormones tend to make skin cells containing dark pigment enlarge, so that any birth mark, freckles, moles or scars tend to become darker after the 3rd month of pregnancy.

These changes mostly disappear after birth, but in some cases they remain. These are normal accompaniments of pregnancy and therefore no cause for worry.

BREAST CHANGES

Breasts often become tender and sensitive to touch in early pregnancy. The tenderness passes by middle pregnancy.

The dark area around the nipple, the areola, gets darker. This is a permanent change in most women.

Stretch marks on the breasts may occur in women with large, heavy or sagging breasts. Hence, you must wear a well-fitting cotton bra, that supports the weight of the breasts. (A nylon bra tends to sag with the weight.) This will not only prevent stretch marks, but prevent sagging too.

VARICOSE VEINS

These are dark, swollen veins that might appear on the legs during pregnancy, and sometimes remain forever afterwards.

The veins in the legs do the job of carrying impure blood back to the heart for purification. In some women the veins become lax or weak during pregnancy. Due to this laxity they cannot push back the blood through the congested pelvic area, so that the blood tends to pool in the legs, causing the appearance of varicose veins.

To prevent their appearance, avoid standing for long periods without moving. Do not cross your legs when sitting on a chair, since this reduces circulation in the legs. Put your feet up on a stool whenever possible. At least once in the day, place your legs higher than your hips. Sit on a chair, put your feet on the table. Or, lying down on the floor, place your feet on a stool, low chair or bed. When sitting for long periods, like at a desk, for instance, write alphabets, A, B, C, etc., with your toes in the air.

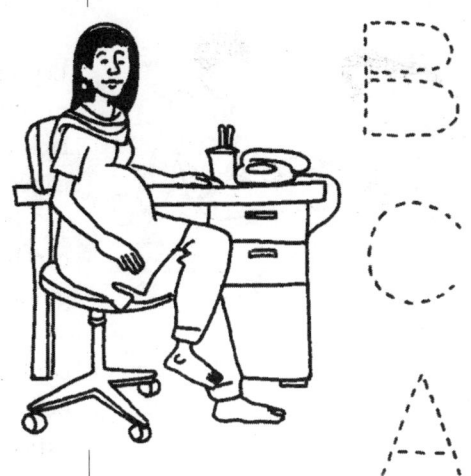

PRECAUTION
Do not point toes if prone to leg cramps. (see p. 54)

TEETH AND GUMS

During pregnancy the gums soften and are therefore more likely to catch infection and start bleeding. Infection in the gums can mean infection in the teeth also, and consequent tooth decay.

Plaque is a layer of bacteria that grows on gums and teeth. Bacteria in plaque thrive on the pieces of food stuck between the teeth, and feed on sugar. If you eat a lot of sugary foods, you increase the amount of plaque in your mouth. If you eat less sugar, the bacteria will not get such a good chance to grow and multiply.

Plaque left on the teeth can eat into the enamel, which is the surface of the tooth. If this is continued, the tooth will keep on decaying until it affects the nerve inside, in the centre of the tooth, causing a toothache.

In order that plaque does not get a chance to form, it is important to brush your teeth regularly and to keep your mouth clean. The good old Indian habit of swishing the mouth a few times with fresh water after a meal is advisable. That apart, brush before sleeping. The best thing is to brush when you know there is going to be a long gap before the next time you eat.

In pregnancy your gums and teeth are in a more delicate condition, so a soft brush is preferred to a hard one. A brush with a small head will reach all the corners and surfaces of your teeth more easily. Change your toothbrush when the bristles begin to look droopy or flat.

Bits of food left between the teeth can irritate the gums and cause them to bleed. You can visit your dentist if you have bleeding gums. Eat fewer sweets and more of salads and fruits. Try home remedies to keep gums and teeth healthy.

There is an old wives' tale that for every baby you lose a tooth. This need not be true. Remember that your gums soften, not the teeth. When the body needs extra calcium to form the baby's teeth and bones and there is not enough in the mother's body, the womb will steal from the mother's bones, making them brittle. The teeth themselves are unaffected. They have to be protected by proper cleanliness.

HOME REMEDIES

After a meal, rinse your mouth with warm salt water.
Brushing with a twig from a kikar or neem tree can be done once a day. However, if you have fillings in your teeth, a twig might dislodge them.
Another good thing for teeth and gums is a mango leaf. Roll a mango leaf and chew on it for some time. Discard the pulp and most of the juice. With a little of the remaining juice, massage your gums with your fingertip. It will make your gums tighten and your teeth shine. It is perfectly safe for fillings too.

Source: Hansaben Yoga Ashram Santacruz, Mumbai

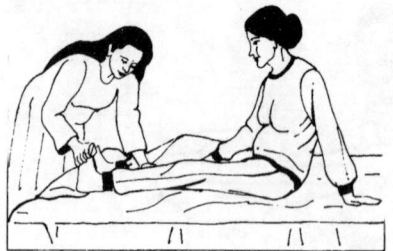

LEG CRAMPS

Leg cramps may occur suddenly in pregnancy and be quite painful. They mostly occur in the last months of pregnancy. Sluggish blood circulation, lack of calcium or magnesium, and lack of Vitamin B or E are thought to cause these cramps.

Point the toes inwards towards the face when the cramp occurs. Someone can hold the painful area of the leg with one hand and with the other hand guide the foot and toes to point towards the face.

Since a change of temperature can also cause a cramp, a hot water bottle could be used in winter to warm your bed. Place a hot water bottle in bed before you go to sleep so that your bed is already warm, and you do not experience the discomfort of getting into a cold bed.

One can increase the intake of milk products, so that the body can get the much needed calcium. Cottage cheese, milk, curds, buttermilk, cheese and greens of radish, turnip, cauliflower, methi, dhania, pudina and all varieties of kerae are good.

Whole and split (chhilka) dals are a good source of Vitamin B. Whole moong, whole masoor, whole urad, split moong and split urad are some examples of this.

Exercising to get the circulation going in the legs should also help. Before sleeping, walk across about a six-foot-long area, on your toes, then on your heels and lastly, on the outer sides of your feet. Done every day before sleeping at night, it has given relief to a lot of women.

Take extra salt, especially at night, in case cramps occur when you are trying to go on a salt-free diet.

SHORTNESS OF BREATH

As pregnancy advances, the uterus presses towards the lungs. This results in shortness of breath and panting, when you climb even a few steps; or the need to take a deep sigh frequently. This is more so in case of a twin pregnancy, or if you are fairly short, so that the uterus feels very large. The discomfort will be more when you sit on something low, when you slump your shoulders or when you lie down. If you sit up straight, it will relieve the discomfort.

It is nothing to worry about; the discomfort will vanish with the birth of the baby.

PALPITATIONS

You might feel that your heart is beating unusually fast. This is called palpitation. Sometimes you might feel your heart is missing a beat. You are more likely to notice this when you exert physically, like walking, climbing stairs, etc. It is quite normal.

It happens because your heart does a lot of extra work when you are pregnant. It needs to pump enough blood around your body to supply both you and your baby with oxygen and nutrients. Also, your blood supply increases in volume by about 40% to keep pace with the increased demands. To cope with this extra volume of blood, the heart actually enlarges, so that it is more powerful. This enables it to pump through the extra blood without speeding up the rate of heartbeat.

Thus it is not surprising to occasionally notice a difference in the way your heart beats. However, palpitations are nothing to worry about.

FAINTING AND DIZZINESS

Because of lowering of blood pressure, not enough oxygen reaches the brain. Sometimes this causes fainting or dizziness. Dizzy spells may also be caused by anaemia.

In the first 3 months of pregnancy the blood pressure is lower than normal. This is why some women complain of dizziness when they first become pregnant. Some of them might actually lose consciousness for a moment or two. This is not harmful to the baby or the mother, except that the mother might injure herself if she falls to the ground in a faint.

In case you have a tendency towards dizzy spells or fainting, avoid crowded and smoky places and long journeys. Avoid moving too suddenly from a lying or sitting position.

ITCHING

Some pregnant women develop an itchy skin, and find red bumps appearing on the abdomen and breasts. This is primarily due to the stretching of the skin and can be aggravated by heavy perspiration or stress. For temporary relief try an oil massage. Women with large breasts often find that it affects them just under the breasts. Calamine lotion may have a soothing effect.

WHEN YOU DO NOT SHOW

The pregnancy does not 'show much' in some pregnant women, who have been athletes, dancers, or who have been exercising regularly or are tall. Their abdomen does not protrude outwards like that of other women in the same month of pregnancy. This is because they have a strong set of healthy muscles. It does not mean that something is wrong with the baby.

STRETCH MARKS

The skin is made up of elastic and non-elastic fibres. When stretching beyond the normal limits occurs, as in pregnancy, the non-elastic fibres tend to break, causing stretch marks. At first these marks may occur as streaks. After birth they take on a kind of purple or brown shade and finally end up as whitish streaks. Excessive water retention (which does not occur as a result of drinking excess water), or weight gain can also cause stretch marks.

These marks may appear on the stomach, breasts, bottom and thighs.

To an extent the marks may be controlled, but cannot be avoided as it is the result of an expanding uterus. Besides, hormonal changes that encourage water retention may cause an increase in fluid retention on your bottom and thighs, causing stretch marks to appear, even in an aware, weight-regulated woman.

The reason why stretch marks are worse in some women is simply that the elasticity of the skin varies from person to person. Women with fewer stretch marks have more elastic fibres in the skin. There is no way in which the skin's elasticity can be increased to reduce stretch marks.

Many women believe that oiling the skin helps, especially with Vitamin E oil. Some women puncture a vitamin E capsule and use it on their bellies. One can never be 100% sure. However, there is no harm in a gentle massage of the stretched abdomen. It is very relaxing. Moreover, if you are lucky, you may find that the marks do not appear at all.

FOOTWEAR

Your feet might swell or fatten further because of the extra weight you now carry. You might need shoes a size larger as compared to what you normally wear. Do not wear high-heeled shoes with heels more than an inch or so high, they will upset your balance, co-ordination, and posture.

Avoid wearing heels during the day and walk barefoot in the evenings at home. All shoes, whether walking shoes or slippers, should have a similar height throughout pregnancy.

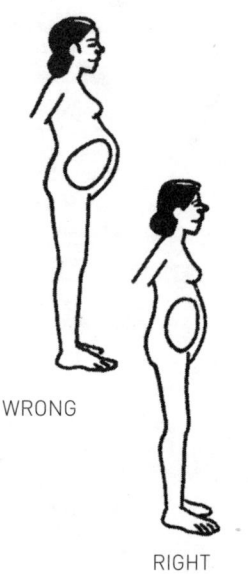

WRONG

RIGHT

NASAL CONGESTION

Mucous membranes inside the nose and sinuses often swell up during pregnancy, on account of certain hormones that also soften up the vagina and the mouth of the womb, in preparation for birth. Some women therefore develop a permanent cold in late pregnancy. However, this will not interfere with your ability to do breathing exercises at the time of labour.

BACKACHE

The weight of the baby is supported by the backbone, with the assistance of the muscles of the back and abdomen. When these muscles are weak, the pressure on the backbone is greater and causes discomfort. When these muscles are strong and toned up, the baby's weight exerts less pressure on the backbone and no backache occurs.

Bad posture also causes backaches. A good posture is simply good balance of the different parts of the body. As you stand, gravity has the effect of constantly pulling you down to the floor, but you remain upright against the force of gravity, by using your muscles to hold yourself erect. If you allow some of your muscles to slacken, other muscles will tighten in order to compensate for the slackening, resulting in bad posture and a strain on your back and other parts of your body.

Typically in pregnancy, one stands with one's bottom out and the hollow of one's back exaggerated. Instead, one should learn to stand straighter. Keep your bottom tucked in and use your abdominal muscles to support the extra weight, instead of overstretching them by just letting them go.

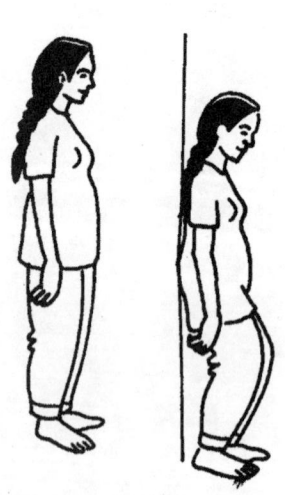

You will benefit by looking and feeling better, and suffering less from backache and tiredness. Also, your stomach will flatten faster after delivery. Tightening your abdominal muscles is not harmful to the baby at all. The baby is comfortably cushioned in the uterus with the amniotic fluid; it gets its supply of oxygen through the umbilical cord; and makes place for itself by nudging the intestines, bladder, liver and other organs away.

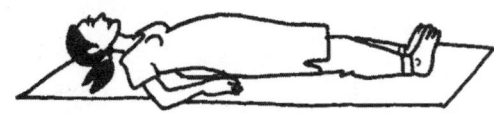

To relieve backaches, pull your tummy in, tuck your bottom in and straighten the length of your backbone against a wall.

Rest should also help soothe your backache. Do not let yourself get overtired. Lie down more often. When lying on your back with legs straight, place a small pillow or folded towel in the hollow of your back.

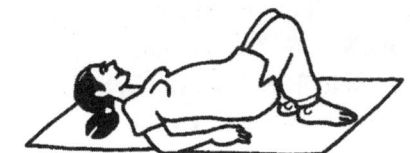

Or else, lie with your legs bent at the knees, feet flat on the floor. As you lie like this, flatten the hollow of your back against the floor.

If you prefer to lie on your side, place pillows as high as your hips. Bend and place the leg on the upper side, bent at the knee, on top of the pile of pillows. Place the arm on the underside, towards your back, along the length of your backbone.

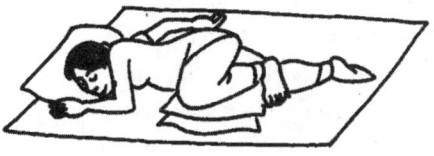

Severe low backache may sometimes be caused by lack of calcium, or by the baby's position. If it is due to lack of calcium, the doctor would recommend supplementary calcium.

Upper backache may be caused by poor posture or heavy breasts. Correct your posture and wear a well-fitting cotton bra, adjusted at the straps to carry the weight of the breasts.

PAIN UNDER THE BREASTS

Pain under the breasts or just below the ribs is common as pregnancy advances, say, after the 8th month. The reason being that, as the baby grows, it extends upwards to below the breasts and tends to push up your organs like the liver, stomach, etc., towards the chest cavity. You will find stretching your arms up, straight above your head, towards the ceiling, helps relieve the discomfort, since it lifts the rib-cage off the growing uterus. Also, sitting straight rather than slouching forward will be more comfortable.

PAIN IN THE GROIN AND SIDES OF ABDOMEN

In late pregnancy it is common to have pain in the pelvic region, since the joints of the pelvic girdle soften in preparation for birth. Avoid standing for a long time. The pain might also result from stretching of the ligaments, which hold the uterus in place.

TINGLING AND NUMBNESS

Tingling and numbness may be felt in the hands in the morning. It is caused by the pressure on the nerves and tendons by the accumulated fluid in hands and wrists. It is felt more in the morning when your wrists have accumulated fluid during the night. To relieve the discomfort, hold your hands above your head for a few minutes and point your fingers towards the ceiling and open and close your fists alternately.

> **NATURAL HEALING**
>
> According to Raikadu Balamma, a popular healer in Pastapur, Andhra Pradesh, oedema can be treated by a handful of crushed fenugreek (methi) leaves and about 10 gm of ginger (adrak), crushed separately. She mixes these to make three tablets. The woman with swelling has to swallow a tablet with water first thing each morning for 3 days. Many women have been cured by this treatment.
>
> *Source:* Touch Me, Touch-Me-Not (Women, Plants and Healing), *published by Kali for Women, 1997*

SWOLLEN HANDS AND FEET

Pregnancy can bring with it swelling of hands, feet, ankles and face. This is called oedema. Since the body retains extra water in pregnancy, a little bit of swelling is normal. Swelling can also be caused by hot weather, tight or ill-fitting shoes or exertion; but this kind of swelling generally disappears during the night, when you are comfortable and it is cooler.

Severe swelling of the hands and feet that does not go away at night could be a symptom of the onset of toxaemia and should be reported to the doctor.

If it occurs, reduce salt intake. Salt encourages retention of water in the body. Avoid foods with a high concentration of salt, e.g. pickles, salted fish, cheese and papad. Also avoid foods high in sugar and carbohydrates e.g. cold drinks, sherbet, juices, chocolates, sweets and reduce consumption of bread, rice, chappatis, pasta.

Eat foods rich in protein e.g. eggs, chickpeas/channa, dal, sprouts, curds, paneer, nuts (see pg. 41).

Avoid standing for long periods of time without rest. Sit whenever possible, and if possible, put your feet up on a stool.

BEHAVIOURAL CHANGES

ABNORMAL CRAVINGS

Desire for abnormal foods like coal and soil is called pica. Generally it is due to lack of minerals like iron or calcium in the body. It was more common in the past. Any leaning towards pica should be dealt with by a correction of deficiencies. Your doctor will tell you what your body misses and how you can correct it.

It should not be confused with a desire for a particular kind of food, like chocolates, in pregnancy. That is, preference for a particular food should not be made an excuse for eating an excess of fattening and sweet things, since heavy food always leads to over weight, which is always considered a health risk.

TIREDNESS

Tiredness is a sign that you need to slow down and take it easy. Try and get at least 10 hours of sleep daily. If you cannot manage it at night, sleep a few hours in the afternoon. Also try and go to bed sooner at night.

In some cases, tiredness may be caused by anaemia (see p. 37).

MOOD SWINGS

Mood swings are common in pregnancy owing to the hormonal changes associated with it. Normally stable women might find themselves going through periods of depression, with tears just beneath the surface. Or a woman might feel high one moment and low the next moment. Warn your near and dear ones of how you feel, to avoid misunderstandings. Strive to be happy and joyful so that the baby benefits by experiencing an environment associated with happiness, rather than one associated with sadness or stress.

SLEEPLESSNESS

Stress and worry can cause sleeplessness. If you are worried about your pregnancy or approaching childbirth, discuss it with your spouse or doctor. It is likely that once you have voiced them, the worries will disappear.

At times although sleep comes to you when you retire to bed at night, you may be woken up in a few hours by a desire to pass urine or by the baby kicking. Thereafter it may be difficult to go back to sleep.

Restrict your fluid intake at night or in the late evening. Try not to worry too much about not being able to go back to sleep. Recite a prayer or a poem in your mind, or, your favourite song. Avoid coffee in the evening, as it is a mild stimulant and might keep you awake at night.

A cup of hot milk just before retiring to bed will help you to relax. A warm salt water bath is also relaxing. Try and consciously relax by doing some deep breathing or the yogic shavasana, the corpse pose.

If you sleep in the afternoons, it would help if you stopped your afternoon nap, so that you can sleep better at night. Instead of a nap in the afternoon you could just relax for about half an hour with music or a book, putting your feet up as you do so.

MEDICINES

Avoid taking medicines on your own. Whatever medicine you take should only be under your doctor's supervision, after you have informed the doctor of your pregnant condition, Indiscriminate use of certain medicines or drugs can harm the baby. It is best to keep drug intake to the minimum.

TRAVELLING

Travelling is no cause for worry if the pregnancy has been normal and stable. Travelling long distances is better done by train than by car or bus. Sitting for long periods should be avoided, since it causes congestion in the legs and pelvic region. In a train, movement is possible and therefore, the discomfort is reduced. Also, a pregnant woman has the need to empty her bladder frequently.

Autorickshaws are safe if you are used to them. But avoid long, bumpy autorickshaw rides on rough roads. On a long, bumpy route, take a bus for most of the journey and an autorickshaw for a small part of it. Request the driver to drive slowly.

If you have high blood pressure or if you have had a miscarriage or bleeding at the beginning of your pregnancy, then travelling by air, even in late pregnancy is not advisable, since the change in altitude may cause premature labour.

Even in a perfectly normal pregnancy, avoid travelling great distances by air in the last 6 weeks, for instance, travelling across time zones. In the last 4 weeks you must remain close to your home and hospital.

Flying in an unpressurised aircraft can cause serious oxygen deprivation to the baby in the first 3 months. However, all modern passenger aircrafts are properly pressurised.

SMOKING

Research has shown that smoking has a marked negative effect on the baby. Smoking after the 4th month of pregnancy causes mental and physical retardation in later childhood, i.e. retardation in the child's reading ability and in its skeletal growth.

Smoking is known to reduce the size of the baby and therefore its chances of survival. Also, smokers lack Vitamin B12, since it is used by the liver to detoxify the effects of smoking.

Smoking reduces the oxygen supply to the baby by causing constriction of the vessels in the placenta, causing intra-uterine growth restriction in the fetus. Even passive smoking, that is, inhaling smoke by sitting in a smoke-filled room, or the husband smoking in the presence of the wife in the bedroom, has the same effect.

Smoking has also been associated with intra-uterine death, premature delivery and rupture of membranes. There is a doubled risk of early spontaneous abortion, stillbirth, congenital abnormality, neonatal death, pre- and post- delivery haemorrhage.

Most women who smoke find that they dislike the taste of cigarettes at the start of pregnancy. It is good for a woman to stop smoking as soon as she finds that she is pregnant. Research has shown that the first 3 months are very crucial, and women should not smoke during this time.

Smoking should be given up totally by women suffering from kidney disease, high blood pressure, pre-eclampsia and bleeding at any stage of pregnancy; also by women who have lost a baby in the first 2 weeks of its life and who have delivered a stillborn child. Smoking would interfere with the development and function of the placenta, so that adequate nourishment and oxygen would not reach the fetus.

Cigarette smoke contains 2 harmful substances, nicotine and carbon monoxide—which do a lot of damage. Nicotine reduces blood supply to the baby, and carbon monoxide, which is like poison, enters the baby's circulation because the baby's blood pigment has a strong affinity for it.

TOBACCO CHEWING

Many people chew tobacco either in a paan (betel leaf) or plain. Tobacco leads to contractions of the blood vessels, so that blood circulation in the uterus and the placenta is impaired. Tobacco consumption during pregnancy diminishes birth weight and length of the baby. It also increases the risk of stillbirth.

It is associated with increased loss of the male fetus and increased placental weight.

It has been shown that nicotine (a substance in tobacco) is excreted in breast milk, saliva and urine. Therefore it is also to be avoided when breastfeeding.

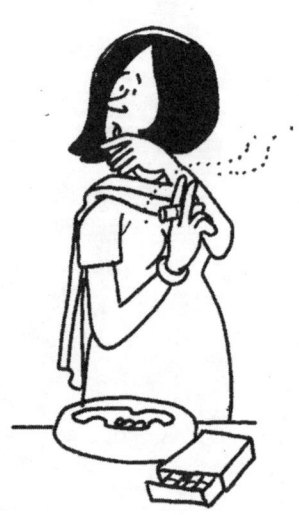

ALCOHOL

Alcohol in pregnancy must be avoided. In the 1960s research began to show that alcohol is teratogenic, that is, capable of causing malformations in the fetus.

Even moderate drinkers can give birth to babies with Fetal Alcohol Syndrome, that is, babies born with jitters, irritability, lethargy and weak sucking reflex.

Parents who consume alcohol can have low birth-weight babies, babies with mental retardation and facial deformities, including flat features and cleft palates.

Even a single heavy-drinking session can impair the growth of a particular organ of the fetus, depending on the stage of development reached at that time.

Since social drinking is common, alcohol does not seem so dangerous, but remember, it is as potent as any drug or medicine taken in the form of a pill. If you are trying to conceive, or if you have just discovered that you are pregnant, cut out alcohol.

Research as to the safe limit of alcohol consumption in pregnancy is continuing. An occasional glass of wine or beer for a perfectly healthy mother may be harmless. Recent research has shown that 25% of women having as little as 2 ounces of alcohol in a week are more likely to have spontaneous abortions as compared to women who do not take alcohol at all.

Alcohol also damages the liver and uses up the B12 vitamin in the body. It is therefore best avoided.

DRIVING

Driving is quite harmless if you remember to drive slowly and carefully. Avoid braking suddenly or any rash driving, since you do not want any mishap.

DIGESTIVE PROBLEMS

VOMITING AND NAUSEA

With pregnancy there is decreased intestinal tone and gastric mobility. This slows down the passage of food through the digestive system and increases the possibility of the absorption of nutrients. On the other hand, it may be one of the factors leading to vomiting in early pregnancy and to constipation in later pregnancy.

Vomiting may also be caused by a rapid rise in hormones in early pregnancy. The level of the hormone gonadotrophin is reduced considerably by the 3rd or 4th month, and this is when a woman tends to feel less sick.

A woman may feel nauseous at any time of the day or night. It usually happens when the stomach is either very empty or very full. So, it makes sense to have 4 moderate meals a day, rather than a heavy lunch and a heavy dinner. Breakfast, lunch, tea and dinner can each be fairly filling, but should not give a stuffed feeling. Or you can have 6 to 7 small meals in a day. You can make sandwiches in advance or keep biscuits, dal sprouts and fruits handy.

HOME REMEDIES

INGREDIENTS: 4 to 5 green cardamoms (small elaichi), 1 black cardamom (big elaichi), 1 tsp aniseed (sauf), the fat variety, ½ cup sugar or mishri or glucose powder.
METHOD: Open up the cardamoms. Heat the tawa or pan, once heated, turn off heat, place the cardamoms and the aniseeds on it and roast lightly. Once roasted, cool and then dry grind. Add to it powdered sugar or mishri. Cool. Bottle.
After a meal have quarter to half a teaspoon for easy digestion.

Nibbling on a biscuit or toast in the morning, before you get out of bed, helps. Also, lying still for about 10 minutes before getting out of bed. Have breakfast 1 hour after waking up.

Avoid tea, coffee, fruit juice, fried and spicy food, and alcohol. Eat a banana between meals.

When you find that you can keep something down, resist eating too much at once. Try eating and drinking things you would not normally eat, in order to find out what you can keep down.

Avoid strong smells. Get someone else to do the cooking. Carbohydrates generally stay down more easily. That is, bread, biscuits, rice, chappatis, potatoes, etc. Do not worry too much about weight gain. Discard tight clothing. Your clothes should be comfortable around the stomach and bust.

Severe vomiting that continues beyond the first 3 or 4 months of pregnancy is called hyperemesis. A woman with hyperemesis is really ill, since she cannot retain any food. Some psychiatrists and obstetricians feel that it is a symptom of disturbed relationships, and if the woman can get away from anyone who is causing her stress, the vomiting will ease off.

It would be a good idea for a woman, who is vomiting at all hours of the day, to get away and live with people she knows slightly. It is a good time to visit an aunt or a relative in another town. The change will settle her down, and she will come back to cope with renewed strength.

Although vomiting does not harm the baby or the pregnancy, in some cases the doctor may recommend hospitalisation. On being admitted the woman will be fed fluids sweetened with sugar or glucose. If the woman has lost a lot of weight, and cannot keep down the fluid she is being fed, she might be put on an intravenous glucose drip. The body needs sugar for its daily requirement. In the absence of adequate intake of sugar the body starts to make acids known as ketones. When these show up in the urine, it is a sign that vomiting is severe and hospitalisation is necessary.

HEARTBURN

This is common from mid-pregnancy onwards. Small amounts of food from the stomach re-enter the food pipe since the stomach valve relaxes and also because of the pressure the growing baby exerts against the stomach. If this happens several times in a day, a burning sensation is felt in the food pipe. To avoid it happening, the stomach should not be completely full or empty. In an empty stomach, acid formation causes this feeling. Sips of cold water should relieve this burning.

To sleep on a full stomach will also cause discomfort. It is a good idea to stay propped up during the night, if it gets very bad. A few extra pillows or cushions will help you stay more upright while you sleep, and it can be quite comfortable. Better still, eat dinner at 7.30 or 8 p.m.

Avoid eating spicy or vinegary foods, excessive salads and green leafy vegetables, and alcohol. Have 4 moderate meals, instead of 2 large meals, in a day.

HOME REMEDIES

A midnight snack is easier to keep down. Keep a snack by your bedside and have it during the course of the night.

FLATULENCE

Flatulence, or wind, is not harmful, but embarrassing. Try keeping away from company when you are passing wind. Avoid gaseous foods like beans, peas, rich food, and excessive amounts of greens.

CONSTIPATION AND PILES

In pregnancy a muscle-relaxing hormone, called relaxin, is secreted by the body, which relaxes, among other things, the digestive system. Relaxing of the digestive system leads to its sluggishness. It therefore requires greater amounts of bulk in it, so as to aid the movement of food through the alimentary canal. Constipation is therefore common in pregnancy.

If you find that you have developed a tendency towards constipation, eat less bread, rice and maida. Eat more chappatis, preferably made of unsieved flour, and pulses or dals. Increase the intake of fruits, salads, vegetables and water.

Bhindi or lady's fingers can be eaten. Dried figs (anjir) are also very good, and easily available at dry-fruit shops. An increase in fluid intake helps, so drink more water. Drink 2 glasses of water on waking up in the morning.

Isabgol (fleaseed husk) can be taken regularly. It is available in packets at chemists' shops. Follow the instructions on the packet. Avoid allopathic laxative pills.

If constipation lingers over a period and is not treated, it can cause veins around the anus to protrude, from straining that accompanies constipation, leading to piles or permanently protruding veins around the anus.

If piles occur, keep constipation in check and avoid spicy food.

DIARRHOEA

This sometimes occurs in pregnancy and it should be reported to the doctor if it persists for more than a day or two. Iron tablets can cause it in some women. In such cases it can be remedied by simply changing the brand of the tablets.

Many women who add lots of fruits and vegetables to their diet find that their stool is a little loose or that they pass stool twice in a day. This should not be confused with diarrhoea.

URINARY TRACT INFECTION

FREQUENT URINATION

In pregnancy one urinates more often as the growing uterus puts pressure on the bladder and restricts the space normally reserved for the storage of urine. The problem will stay until the birth of the baby. At the most you can limit the intake of fluids in the evening, so that you do not have to wake up at night too often to go to the toilet.

HOME REMEDIES

In case of diarrhoea, having a mixture of black tea and a slightly overripe mashed banana helps. One could put the mashed banana in a soup bowl and pour black tea over it. Cool it before having it.

URINARY TRACT INFECTION

An infection in the urinary tract causes inflammation of the bladder and urethra, the pipe through which urine is passed. This is called cystitis. Cystitis is a common complaint that could occur in pregnancy.

The first symptom is usually the desire to pass urine more frequently, sometimes only minutes after having already done so. Most of the time you will not be able to pass much urine, perhaps only a trickle or not at all. This can be accompanied by a burning sensation or stinging. When you do manage to pass some urine, it may be very dark yellow in colour, and in extreme cases, streaked with blood.

This infection is easily caused in women because of the female anatomy; since the openings of the urethra, vagina and anus are all very close together. Germs from the stool get transmitted very easily to the urethra and vagina.

CYSTITIS

It is important to consult your doctor as soon as possible if you have an attack of cystitis, because if it is left untreated the infection can travel to the kidney and be very painful and dangerous. Cystitis is very easily treated, once diagnosed early. A course of antibiotics will soon rid the infection.

To relieve the symptoms of cystitis immediately, drink a glass of water every half hour, to dilute the strength of the urine, and to help flush the infection through, before it gets a chance to take hold. Any watery liquid will do, for example, a lemon or barley drink, weak tea, lassi, etc. This helps make the urine less acidic (alkaline urine is inhospitable to germs) and therefore less painful when passed.

If you have suffered from cystitis several times before, and think you may be prone to developing the infection again, there are 2 things you can do to lessen the likelihood of an attack. First, drink plenty of fluids. It is a good idea to make it a habit to drink 2 glasses of water on waking up in the morning. It will also help relieve constipation. Second, be more hygienic. Every time you pass stool, wash the anal area not only with water, but with soap and water; and do not bring your hand forward towards your urethra as you do so. Better still, wash from behind. During your bath, use soap and water to wash the vaginal area. Similarly, wash your anus separately.

VAGINAL DISCHARGE

It is normal to have increased vaginal discharge in pregnancy, because the glands at the mouth of the womb increase their output.

The discharge is actually cleansing the vagina and keeping it free of infection, as well as lubricating the tissues of the vagina as they become thicker, softer, and more elastic in preparation for birth. During subsequent pregnancies the discharge will be less. Make sure you wear cotton underwear to allow your skin to breathe.

If you notice a change in the discharge from white to yellow or green, and if it causes itching or irritation, becomes thicker or smells unpleasant, you probably have an infection. It is a minor, harmless infection called thrush, Candida or monilia.

It is easily treated with creams or pessaries, under the doctor's guidance. Sometimes the pessaries may be supplemented with antibiotics. Early treatment is desirable to prevent future complications.

During the advanced stage of pregnancy, that is, if your baby is due within a month and you have a discharge that looks like the beginning of a period, a thick mucus discharge, tinted with dried blood (pink or brown), it is a sign that your body is getting ready for birth. Take it as a signal. It is just that, and not an emergency.

CONDITIONS NEEDING SPECIAL ATTENTION

VAGINAL BLEEDING

In early pregnancy, vaginal bleeding may be caused because the level of your pregnancy hormone is not sufficiently high to stop your period. The bleeding will be scanty and it will occur when a period would have been due. Such bleeding is not a miscarriage. The doctor may give an injection of progesterone hormone or advise bed rest.

Sometimes a few drops of blood may appear after intercourse, or a vaginal examination by the doctor.

Late in pregnancy, bright-red bleeding, like that which flows at the height of a period, is serious, although quite rare. It can be caused by the placenta, the organ that nourishes the baby, detaching from the wall of the uterus. The seriousness will depend on how large a portion of the placenta has separated from the uterus. The doctor should be informed immediately.

You might be advised to go to the hospital for bed rest. Lying down increases the blood flow to the uterus and if the placenta is not firmly rooted, gives it a chance to root itself firmly to the wall of the uterus. If bleeding stops and all is well with the baby, you will be permitted to go home in a few days. In this case it is wise to avoid intercourse and orgasm until after the baby is born.

Sometimes bleeding is caused by the placenta lying too low between the baby's head and the mouth of the womb. This is called placenta previa and means delivery by Caesarean section in case of placenta previa major i.e. if the placenta is centrally covering the mouth of the womb. It could also mean bed rest, at home or hospital, before the birth of the baby. If the placenta only reaches towards the mouth of the uterus, it often shifts and moves away as the pregnancy advances and the uterus grows and stretches. It is possible in such cases to have a normal delivery.

HIGH BLOOD PRESSURE

Any physical movement such as running or jumping can temporarily raise the blood pressure, but it returns to normalcy after a period of rest.

Excessive weight gain could raise blood pressure. Also, a stressful lifestyle, or a nervous, easily agitated and highly strung person, tends to be prone to high blood pressure.

It is therefore important to rest when you feel you are getting tired and tense. Avoid unnecessary nerve-racking activity, like watching a late night horror/violent movie.

Rising blood pressure will be a cause for concern to your doctor. At every visit to your doctor, the blood pressure is measured, the reason being that rising blood pressure could herald the beginning of certain complications of pregnancy, such as toxaemia, which need special attention and care.

If the diastolic blood pressure (the lower figure of the recorded level, e.g. 120/70) rises by as much as 20, you are considered to have high blood pressure or hypertension. Bed rest will be prescribed, since the placenta will work more efficiently if you stay in bed. In late pregnancy, many obstetricians induce labour if the diastolic reading of your blood pressure rises to 90 or above.

If you have high blood pressure, try taking a warm bath before going to bed at night. It will help you relax and sleep better.

TOXAEMIA AND PRE-ECLAMPSIA

TOXAEMIA: WHEN RINGS DO NOT FIT

Toxaemia usually occurs only during the last few weeks of pregnancy and is recognised by 3 typical symptoms. Any of these symptoms appearing by itself does not mean you have toxaemia. It is only when they appear together that they spell toxaemia. The first symptom is increased blood pressure. The second sign is swelling of hands, feet and face the third sign is the appearance of protein in the urine.

These are warning signals. If they are not heeded, convulsions may occur. The toxaemia has then become a serious condition known as eclampsia.

Vigilant pre-natal health care can prevent this condition or make it less serious. Once a woman is excreting a high proportion of protein in her urine, pregnancy is not likely to continue for longer than 2 weeks.

A well-balanced diet, with more protein and less carbohydrate and salt, reduces the incidence of toxaemia. Rest will also help.

If symptoms continue, the woman is usually put into a hospital for further treatment, and if necessary, early delivery of the baby. However, once the condition is identified, complete bed rest in hospital with careful monitoring of the symptoms is usually enough to prevent it from getting worse.

Toxaemia can harm the unborn baby. If it progresses unchecked, it can cause the placenta to fail, and lead to premature labour before the baby is mature enough to survive. When toxaemia becomes eclampsia, it can cause fits and coma. The following are signs of eclampsia: headache, flashing lights, nausea, vomiting and pain in the abdomen.

Toxaemia and eclampsia should not be taken lightly. Starting as a minor ailment they can develop into a dangerous disease.

ANAEMIA

In pregnancy, blood tests are taken to find out the haemoglobin content. Haemoglobin is present in the red blood cells, and is the means by which oxygen is conveyed from the lungs to the cells in the body, including the baby in the womb. If there is not enough haemoglobin in the mother's blood, there may not be enough oxygen reaching the baby for its optimum growth and development.

However, haemoglobin levels tend to drop in pregnancy, because the fluid volume of the mother's blood increases, and thinner blood makes more fluid-carrying nutrients become available to the baby. If the haemoglobin falls below 9 gms/100 ml, a woman is considered anaemic.

A woman who is anaemic feels tired, exhausted, irritable, lethargic, weak and over worked, even though she may be doing little physical work. She might also experience shortness of breath and dizzy spells.

If a woman is found to be anaemic, she should increase her daily intake of iron, until the required haemoglobin level is reached. This can be done by taking a course of iron tablets, and by adding iron-rich foods in the diet.

Foods rich in iron are green cauliflower leaves, mustard leaves or sarson, leafy greens, ganth gobhi or knol khol greens, mint or pudina, dhania or coriander leaves, jaggery, eggs, etc. Although spinach has iron, most of it cannot be used by the body, because other substances present in spinach block absorption of iron by the blood.

If a woman avoids putting on too much weight in pregnancy, she will need less haemoglobin to sustain her body. Unnecessary weight gain requires extra blood, haemoglobin, oxygen and nutrients, thus overworking all the mechanisms of the body. Hence, excessive weight gain always works to your disadvantage.

RHESUS-NEGATIVE

All blood is either rhesus-negative or rhesus-positive. You run a risk only if you have a rhesus-negative blood group while your husband has a rhesus-positive blood group. A routine blood test at the beginning of the pregnancy will show whether you are rhesus-positive or negative. There is no symptom of rhesus incompatibility that you will notice.

If you are a rhesus-negative mother bearing a rhesus-positive baby some of the baby's red cells may leak into your blood circulation. This is most likely in late pregnancy or at the time of delivery. Your body responds to the baby's blood as it would to an invader and your natural defence mechanisms will produce antibodies against it. If these antibodies leak back to the baby's circulation, they can destroy a large number of the baby's blood cells and cause severe anaemia and jaundice in the newborn.

In the first baby there is not enough time for this to happen, since the leak mostly occurs at the time of delivery. But the mother's antibodies can

---

HOME REMEDIES

To increase haemoglobin levels, soak one raisin (kishmish) overnight in water. In the morning boil it in a cup of milk, then drink the milk and eat the raisin. On day two soak 2 raisins overnight in water. In the morning boil them in a cup of milk, then drink the milk and eat the raisins. Likewise go on to 3, 4, 5, 6, 7, 8 and finally 9 raisins. Then go back to 8, 7, 6, 5, 4, 3, 2, and finally one raisin.

On completion of 18 days your haemoglobin level is likely to rise.

Source: Anand P. Verma, Accupressurist

damage the blood cells of any rhesus-positive baby carried by the mother in future. The antibodies can vigorously attack the baby's blood so that the baby might get anaemia, jaundice or brain damage and may not survive.

In order to avoid this happening, an injection of anti-D immunoglobulin can be given to a rhesus-negative mother in pregnancy or immediately after the birth of a rhesus-positive baby. This injection is a serum which is to be given within 48 hours after the birth of a baby. It stops the mother's biological defence mechanism from acting against the foreign rhesus substances. A fresh injection is given after every delivery, miscarriage or abortion. It is possible for blood from an aborted fetus to enter the mother's bloodstream.

GERMAN MEASLES, RUBELLA

This is a mild but very infectious disease that lasts a few days. It is caused by a virus and may cause a slight rash and fever, sometimes accompanied by swollen glands and aching joints. On the other hand, it may go unnoticed. The rash is the main sign, and lasts only 12 to 24 hours. If you fail to see a doctor when the rash occurs, a blood test taken 2 weeks later will show a highlevel of antibodies from recent infection and confirm the diagnosis.

Rubella has grave consequences for the unborn child. If you suffer from it in the first 3 months of pregnancy it may cause deafness, blindness, and congenital heart disease or any other type of abnormality. Later in pregnancy the risk is much less, and could be restricted to deafness. The virus may also cause a miscarriage, low birth-weight baby or stillbirth. If you catch rubella in the first 3 months of pregnancy, your doctor will advise a medical termination of pregnancy.

If you have been in contact with someone who has measles or has recently had measles, or who develops measles within 2 or 3 days of seeing you, consult your doctor. A couple of blood tests done 2 weeks apart will help the doctor decide whether the pregnancy should be continued or terminated.

Do not be shy in avoiding relatives or friends when they have measles in the house. Tell them it is doctor's orders. Absent yourself from your place of work if there is measles there.

Mothers should immunise their daughters against rubella when they are around 10 to 14 years of age.

If you are not sure whether you have had rubella, a blood test for rubella antibodies will make it clear. If a blood test shows that you have never had rubella, you can be immunised after your baby is born, to avoid worry in future. However, the inoculation should not be taken during pregnancy, and once taken in the non-pregnant state, conception should be avoided for the next 3 months.

DIABETES

Diabetes mellitus is a disorder of sugar metabolism. In a normal person the pancreas produce the hormone insulin, this helps to absorb glucose from the bloodstream.

In a diabetic person the pancreas produce insufficient insulin or the insulin produced does not do its job properly, causing the sugar levels in the person's blood and urine to become abnormally high.

A pregnant diabetic woman may be diabetic before pregnancy or may develop diabetes during pregnancy, called 'gestational diabetes'.

Those who were already diabetic need to talk to a specialist before becoming pregnant. During pregnancy they need a careful working out of the dosage of the medicine that they require to take, and to regularly monitor their blood sugar.

Most women with gestational diabetes can keep their diabetes under control by reducing the amount of sugar and calories in their diet.

A diabetic woman needs regular antenatal check-ups so that any complication can be dealt with as soon as possible. If there are no complications due to careful diet habits of the mother, and her well-being and that of the baby are carefully monitored, she can easily have a normal delivery.

A mother with diabetes should avoid sweets (sweet drinks and sweet foods), and eat less of carbohydrates. That is, she should eat less of bread, rice, chappatis, potatoes and pasta.

She should eat more protein. If she can have an egg daily it will be good for her and the baby. Vegetarian sources of protein are chana in any form. Chickpeas or Kabuli chana, horse gram or kala chana, chana dal, chickpea flour or besan (dhokla, khandvi, missi roti, besan curry, pakoras) or plain roasted chana are examples.

Nuts are another good source of protein. Almonds or badams, peanuts or moongphali etc. Also high on protein are curd, paneer, lassi, curry made from curd, sprouts. Foods that mix cereals and pulses or lentils are also good.

A mother can have with her meals less of chappatis, rice or bread, and more of curd, cottage cheese or paneer, pulses or dals, lentils or rajma, lobia, and non-vegetarian foods or eggs.

Also, if a mother is diabetic it is a good idea for her to eat salad before her meal. She should have a quarter plate full of salad—tomatoes, cucumber, onion, radish, carrot, salad leaves, whatever she fancies.

Also see pg. 90

5

*We may live without books—
what is knowledge but
grieving?
We may live without hope—
what is hope but deceiving?
We may live without passion—
what is passion but pining?
But where is the man that can
live without dining?*

Owen Meredith

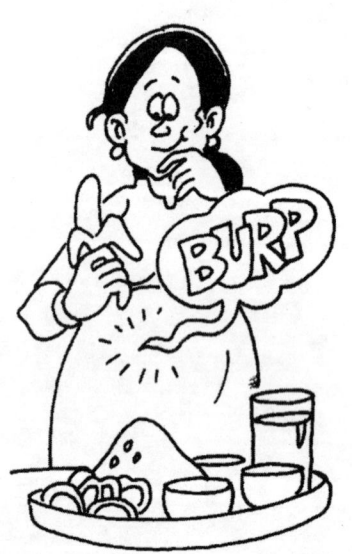

DIET IN PREGNANCY AND AFTER

EATING FOR TWO

There is a common belief that a pregnant woman should eat for 2 people. This is not necessary, but it is essential to eat the right food. One needs to eat nutritious food. Everything that you eat should have good food value, that is, one should eat wisely to nourish yourself and the baby; but not twice as much.

A PARASITE

The baby takes the nutrients it requires, regardless of whether you have enough or not. It takes, for instance, enough iron to store in its liver for the first 3 months of its life, not to mention the iron it uses up for the formation of its blood.

Then it takes calcium from your body to form its bones and the foundation of its teeth. If you do not consume enough calcium, it is going to take calcium away from your bones. You cannot afford to let this happen, for you will need good health and strength to look after your baby after it is born. So you must make it a point to eat well.

FOODS YOU NEED

The foods you need to eat are those rich in iron, calcium and proteins.

IRON

Iron is present in green leafy vegetables. It is a good idea to keep *pudina* or *dhania* (mint or coriander) chutney handy. Make small quantities of it and store in a covered bottle in the refrigerator. Prepare it every 3rd or 4th day. Two teaspoons of chutney a day will meet a good part of your daily iron requirement. You can use it instead of butter to spread on bread when making a sandwich (see p. 37). Iron is also present in kishmish or raisins. It is present in gur or jaggery and powdered brown sugar, which is different from caramelised white sugar. It is present in any dish cooked in an iron pan. However, food cooked in an iron pan becomes black, unless the pan is treated with a thin layer of oil and heated before being used for cooking.

When cooked, remove the food into a stainless steel or glass bowl or else it may turn blackish in colour.

Dried fish is especially rich in both iron and calcium. So are yeast tablets, radish leaves, knolkhol or ganth gobhi leaves, kerai or leafy greens, cauliflower leaves, etc. The iron in spinach is not easily absorbed.

Vitamin C promotes iron absorption. Vitamin C is found in citrus fruits, tamarind or imli; Indian gooseberry or amla; dried raw mango powder or amchur.

Kabuli chana or whole bengal gram, kala chana or horse gram, rajma or kidney beans, sabut moong or green gram are also rich in both iron and calcium.

Also, if you do not sieve the atta or flour before making chapattis you will get iron and Vitamin B from it.

CALCIUM

Calcium is available from milk and milk products. Ideal would be the consumption of about 3 glasses of milk in a day. It can be had in different forms. As curd, cheese, paneer, custard, buttermilk or *lassi*, even curry made from curd.

Calcium is also present in green leafy vegetables. But if you have gas or flatulence, heartburn or sour burps, you should not have too much of green leafy vegetables. About one tablespoon at a time should be easy to digest and not cause a gastric disturbance.

Eggs and lemons are a good source of calcium. Lack of calcium in the long run makes you weak. It can also cause backache or cramps. It causes irritability for its lack causes the nerves to twitch.

Vitamin D promotes calcium absorption. Our body makes Vitamin D when exposed to sunshine (directly on the skin). So expose yourself to the morning sun without wearing sunscreen. The morning sun does not burn. If you worry about your skin burning, use any product with aloe after exposure, for instance, an aloe gel or lacto calamine with aloe.

PROTEIN

Protein is the body's building material. You need protein not only to build a baby's body but also to look after the wear and tear and maintenance of your own body.

If you have an egg a day, and pulses or *dals* with your meals, you should get enough proteins.

However, if you are a pure vegetarian and do not eat eggs at all, you must take care to see that your diet contains adequate protein. *Dals* are a good source of protein, but not the best.

The best vegetarian source is a cereal and pulse mixture. Cereal e.g. wheat or rice combined with pulses or *dal* is a good source of protein. Cereals have a protein that is absent in pulses, and pulses have a protein that is absent in cereals. Combined, they make a good source of protein, each providing an essential protein exclusive to themselves.

Essential amino acids or proteins are those that cannot be manufactured by the body. They are required to be sourced through the diet. Pulses provide the body with the essential amino acid lysine and cereals provide the essential protein methionine. Therefore, vegetarians need to eat a mixture of cereals and pulses.

For non-vegetarians who eat meat at least three times a week, the protein intake is adequate. But if you eat meat only when you eat out or entertaining at parties, you should consider yourself to be a vegetarian.

Another good source of protein is milk and milk products, that is, paneer, curd and so on. Nuts like peanuts or moongphali, almonds or badams, cashewnuts or kajus, walnuts or akhrot and all other nuts, are also a good source of protein. Badam traditionally is considered superior to other nuts, but nutritionally it is of no superior value. Nuts also have a fair amount of fat.

Chana too is a very good source of protein, be it chana dal, besan, or the roasted chana sold by chanawalas. Chana is a good thing to keep handy to eat between meals. You can eat it instead of biscuits or fried namkeen. It will be better for your figure as well as for your nutrition. You can keep chana mixed with little pieces of jaggery in a jar to eat when hungry. While chana will provide you with protein, jaggery will provide you with iron.

Soyabean is an excellent source of protein. However it is not a healthy source of protein for two reasons.

Firstly, it has a high amount of estrogen hormone which pregnant women don't need. Growing children and men also do not need extra female hormone. It can cause the feminization of little boys. In girls it can cause early puberty.

The second reason why soyabean should not be had by anybody, including women after menopause, is; that it is a genetically modified crop.

GENETICALLY MODIFIED CROPS

Genetically modified crops include genes extracted from bacteria, to make the crop resistant to pest attacks. Genetically modified brinjal, whose commercial release was stopped in 2010, has a toxin derived from a soil bacterium called Bacillus thuringiensis (BT).

Till now, scientists and multinational corporations promoting GM crops have maintained that the BT toxin, which is widely used in all GM crops, poses no danger to human health, as the protein breaks down in the intestines of human beings. However, doubts have arisen about the safety of GM crops, since a study reported the presence of BT toxins in human blood.

The first genetically modified soybeans were planted in the U.S. in 1996. In 2007 close to 60% of the world's soyabean crop was genetically modified. The planting of GM soyabean crops has only gone up since then. Today the percentage of GM soyabean crops is 100% in Argentina, 94% in USA. Large-scale commercial planting of GM Soya crops is spreading to many countries.

There are no strict labelling laws as yet to alert the consumer as to whether the ingredients in food are genetically modified or not. It is best to avoid packed foods or food supplements that have soya as one of the ingredients.

In Europe soya is used to feed livestock, that is, pigs, cows, chickens, etc. to be eventually eaten as meat.

Soya oil is extracted and refined and sold in the market as cooking oil.

Soya is also used to produce numerous food ingredients and additives. Lecithin, for example, is used as an emulsifier in chocolate, ice-cream, margarine and baked goods like bread.

Soy milk is also available in the market. Tofu and soy sauce are other soya products.

Some energy bars, packed diet foods, namkeen, biscuits, food supplements also contain soya.

According to *The Guardian* (August 2002), a study shows the disadvantages of GM foods for human health.

British scientific researchers demonstrated that genetically modified DNA from crops can find its way into human gut (intestinal) bacteria, raising possible health concerns. This is because antibiotic-resistance marker genes are inserted with GM material, which could cause a person to be resistant to antibiotic medicines.

Michael Antonio, a senior lecturer in molecular genetics at King's College Medical School, London, said, 'Research suggests that antibiotic marker genes could spread around the stomach and compromise antibiotic resistance. If this were to happen, a person could be immune to beneficial antibiotic medicines'.

The House of Lords has called for them to be phased out as swiftly as possible. The research was conducted at the request of the UK's Food Standards Agency.

Scientists from the University of Sherbrooke, Canada, have detected the insecticidal protein, Cry1Ab, circulating in the blood of pregnant as well as non-pregnant women.

The presence of Cry1Ab was detected in blood samples taken before delivery from pregnant women, and at tubal ligation from non-pregnant women. It was also found in fetal blood from samples taken from the umbilical cord after birth, implying that it could pass on to the next generation. The research paper has been peer-reviewed and accepted for publication in the journal, *Reproductive Toxicology*.

The women that were tested were all consuming food typically being consumed in Canada. Their diet included GM foods such as soybean, corn and potatoes. It can also pass to humans through consumption of meat where the animals have been fed GM foods in livestock feeds.

Governments have encouraged GM foods in the hope of making it easier to feed millions. Since these foods do not spoil easily, it is easy to store them.

However, the very factors that make the shelf life of these foods longer are what are extremely harmful to human health. It was earlier believed that they would be de-activated in the human digestive tract. But this has not happened, as recent research is proving. It is not worth sacrificing health to be able to consume plenty. It is better to eat less, but eat healthy. Healthy food also gives satisfaction or satiety; you therefore do not need to eat huge quantities of it.

In India genetically modified crops so far have been brinjal and cotton. However GM brinjal was discontinued.

Since cotton seed oil is used in India, toxins may have already entered the food chain. It is best to avoid all genetically modified crops.

Organic foods are a little more expensive but good for your health.

- There is a very interesting book called *Food Rules* by Michael Pollan (Penguin Books) that guides you on how to eat healthy. It is a highly recommended book. I am writing here some helpful tips on healthy eating. To understand these points further, you need to read the book.
- Eat food. Not too much. Mostly plants.
- If it came from a plant, eat it. If it was made in a plant, don't.
- Eat only foods that will eventually rot, (It means that food is alive. Only alive things die. Synthetic things do not die. Plastic, for instance.)
- Avoid products that make health claims.
- Avoid foods that are pretending to be something they are not. Example, imitation butter i.e. margarine, mock meats, artificial sweeteners, fake fats and starches.

Eat foods you can picture in their raw state or growing in Nature.

WHOLESOME FOODS

A cereal, pulse and vegetable mixture makes a very wholesome meal. For example, dosa or idli with sambhar and coconut chutney.

Another such combination can be made with parathas. If you make a dough of half besan or chickpea flour and half wheat flour and add to it chopped radish or mooli leaves, it will make quite a wholesome meal. Also, a paratha made of mixed flour of wheat, horse gram or kala chana and barley or jowar with radish or other green leaves of mint, coriander or any other chopped in it, is good. One can use green leaves of spring onions, mustard/sarson, fenugreek/methi, kerai, etc. These parathas are a meal in themselves and can be eaten with curd for breakfast, lunch, or dinner.

Pickles have a high concentration of salt and are to be avoided if you are getting swollen hands and feet. Butter should be avoided if you are overweight.

Another nutritious food is sprouted whole dals (e.g. whole green gram dal/sabut moong dal), or lentils (e.g. horse gram/kala chana). They are best eaten raw. Cooking reduces their food value, by destroying Vitamins B and C. However, their protein value is not destroyed by cooking. To make them at home, clean, wash and soak the *dal* or lentils for at least 4-5 hours in summer and 8-10 hours in winter. You could soak them overnight. Then wash with water and place in a small flat-bottomed steel vessel. Cover the vessel with a lid which you leave slightly open for air.

After 6 to 9 hours toss the lentils or pulses so that the ones on the bottom of the vessel come to the top and the lentils or pulses on the top go down. Pour a little water to moisten it. If the water is in excess, drain it out and leave it semi-covered again. Repeat till the sprouts are the length you would like them.

FOLLOWING IS THE LIST OF 5 FOOD SECTIONS ON
THE PYRAMID STARTING WITH HEALTHY FOODS.

Fresh seasonal fruits and vegetables, lemons, raw nuts, green chutney, tender coconut water, piece of coconut, betel leaf/paan, curry leaves/kari patta, seeds like til (sesame), alsi (flaxseed), seeds of melons, pumpkin, cucumber, amaranth/chaulai/ramdana, organic foods

Pulses or dals, lentils (rajma, chana, lobia), milk and milk products (dahi, paneer, chach, khoya), well-cooked eggs and meats, oats, African finger millet/ragi/nachni/maduva/bavto/marwa/kayappi/taidalu/panjapulle; idli & sambhar, khichdi & dahi, brown rice.

Chappati, rice, porridge (dalia), bread, pasta, pakoras, cheese, ice-cream, kulfi

Butter, cream, pastries, chocolates, mathis, jalebis.

Excess of salt, sugar or refined flour/maida, jams and preservatives, pickles, cold drinks, aerated drinks, ready to eat packed foods, high fructose corn syrup, ajinomoto/MSG/mono sodium glutamate/E 621; raw eggs, chemicals (preservatives), GM crops

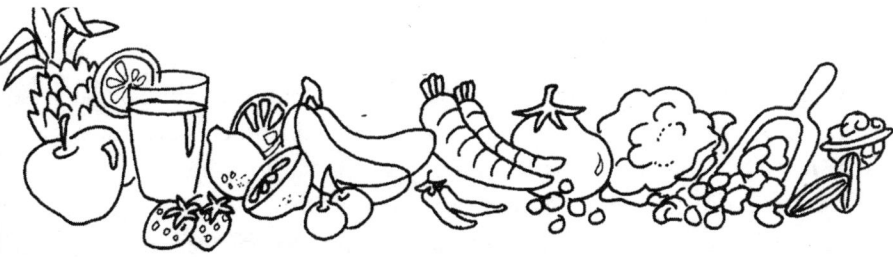

They can be added to chopped salad, to cucumber cubes or grated radish. They can be sprinkled on vegetables or added to sandwich fillings. They can be made into a savoury by themselves, by adding lemon juice, chopped onions, coriander, green chillies and salt.

Potato is a highly misunderstood vegetable. Although potatoes do have carbohydrates, they are 99.9% fat-free and 100% cholesterol-free. They have vitamins B and C, and some proteins. Boiled potatoes are a good and cheap source of nutrition. Potatoes become fattening only when they are fried. At tea time one can have boiled potatoes with salt, chopped onions, lemon juice and chopped mint or coriander leaves added to them. Potatoes contain more moisture or water than cereals; therefore they contain fewer calories as compared to cereals.

If you keep boiled potatoes in the fridge, they can be handy when you need a quick bite, but lack the time to cook. Do not skin or cut potatoes before you boil them; that way they lose nutrition. Boil them in their jackets. When boiled, the skin should not break.

Then there is the highly recommended category of seasonal fruits and vegetables. Guavas, oranges, watermelons, and bananas. Cucumbers and carrots eaten raw will give you vitamins and minerals.

TEA, COFFEE AND COLA DRINKS AND CHOCOLATES

Excessive amounts of tea, coffee, cola drinks and chocolates should be avoided. They contain caffeine and other related substances like tannic acid, which impair and upset digestion.

Caffeine is a diuretic, that is, it causes more urine to be passed. This also washes away essential salts and water soluble vitamins. Further, it reduces absorption of iron and calcium. It can also cause sleep disturbances, anxiety and heartburn.

The amount of caffeine present in a cup of tea or coffee depends on the quality used and the amount of time taken to brew it. The more bitter it is, the more the caffeine content.

TO AVOID PUTTING ON TOO MUCH WEIGHT

You must make sure you do not eat out of compulsion when you get tense. Instead, have a warm water bath with a spoonful of salt added to it. It is very relaxing. Or, start some activity like tidying your cupboard, baking a cake, embroidery, making pickles, etc.

Avoid white sugar as far as possible. Palm sugar and sugar made from powdered jaggery have nutritional elements in them; but white sugar is so overprocessed that 99% of its non-carbohydrate constituents are taken away from it, and it ends up as a plain energy-giving carbohydrate.

Sugar is quickly digested, and is readily absorbed by the body, giving a tremendous lift of energy. This lift lasts until the sugar gets used up, and immediately one feels like eating something sweet again, to get over the low feeling that follows. So you develop a sweet tooth. What you do is that you inhibit the body's ability to produce the necessary energy from all other food. The body takes energy from sugar instead and the other energy is converted into fat. This would also apply to women who have several cups of sweet tea or several glasses of cold drinks a day.

METHODS OF COOKING

Steaming is the best method of cooking as loss of nutrients is minimal. Boiling is good only if the water in which food has been boiled is also consumed. Frying, overcooking, and reheating cause a loss of nutrients and are best avoided or kept to a minimum.

If you feel you are developing a sweet tooth, the first thing to do is to have naturally sweet things instead. Example: Jaggery, raisins, mango, chikoo, honey, dates, etc. These sweet things will also give you nutrition, along with sweetness. Avoid chocolates, sweets, lollipops, ice-creams, cakes, pastries, etc. Then switch to substituting a few sweet things with cheese, chana, apple, carrot, cucumber, sprouted moong dal, etc.

Gradually wean yourself away from your addiction for sweet things. Make it a slow but sure process. Be gentle but firm with yourself and you will find that you have retrained your taste buds by the end of it, and your desire for sweets will have diminished.

Do not use sweetex or other sugar substitutes. Remember, you are trying to cultivate a new taste. It is hard to stop craving sugar if you take artificial sweeteners.

Avoid excessive oil in your cooking. Reduce the number of deep-fried things you eat. For example, chips and pakoras, puris, fried namkeen, fried papad, etc. When you have made a vegetable, there should be no oil left in the serving dish after the vegetable has been eaten. If oil remains, it is a sign that the oil used was in excess. Also, when you make curries, there should be no oil floating on the surface of the curry.

Kidney beans or rajma, chickpeas or kabuli chana, horse gram or kala chana, all kinds of pulses can be boiled with salt, turmeric, garam masala, onion, ginger and a teaspoon of oil; and eaten with vegetables and chappatis. Avoid fried masalas in them. Thick rich masala curries are fattening. So are white sauce, thick soup, mayonnaise and foods laced with creamy sauces. All highly refined foods should be avoided, because most of the goodness or nutrition has been taken away from them. Maida and sugar-based foods would come under this category; for example, samosas, cakes, noodles, white bread, jalebis, jams, rice, kachoris, mathris, etc.

Interestingly, khoya, besan and paneer-based Indian sweets also give protein, apart from sugar. For instance, Bengali mithai, besan ladoos, rasgullas, chenna murgi, barfi, patisa are some examples.

If you tend to eat a lot at meals, fill yourself with lassi, raw vegetables or fruit. Do not add ghee to your dal or chappatis.

BODY WEIGHT

How much weight should a woman put on in pregnancy is a matter of great interest and controversy. Earlier the permitted weight was 9 to 10 kg. Then it became 12.5 kg and now it is accepted that it may be a little higher than 12.5 kg.

If at the start of pregnancy you were underweight, you can take the advantage of putting on more weight than a woman who started pregnancy being overweight. If you have a tendency to gain weight more rapidly than other women, you will have to be careful with the weight increase.

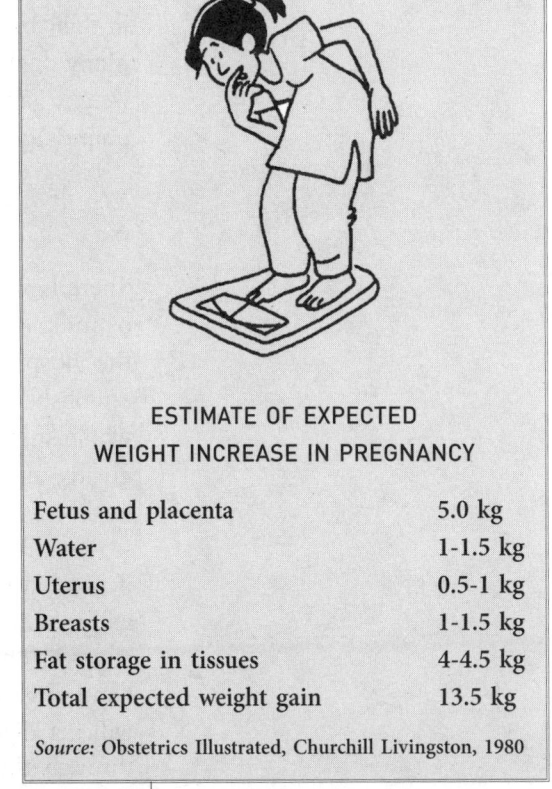

ESTIMATE OF EXPECTED WEIGHT INCREASE IN PREGNANCY

Fetus and placenta	5.0 kg
Water	1-1.5 kg
Uterus	0.5-1 kg
Breasts	1-1.5 kg
Fat storage in tissues	4-4.5 kg
Total expected weight gain	13.5 kg

Source: Obstetrics Illustrated, Churchill Livingston, 1980

> **PERCENTAGE WEIGHT INCREASE DURING PREGNANCY**
>
> On an average a woman puts on a total of 25% of her non-pregnant weight.

One thing is for sure, pregnancy is not a time to diet or try and remain slim. You need a variety of foods to nourish yourself and the baby.

All the weight you put on is not added to you, it is needed by your body to support and nourish the baby. After birth, a lot of fat laid down in the tissues is used up to breastfeed the baby. Women who do not feed their babies find it difficult to lose the weight they put on in their tissues; typically on their hips, upper back, thighs and upper arms.

In the first 3 months of pregnancy there may not be any weight gain. Weight might actually fall as a result of nausea, vomiting and loss of appetite. Gain in weight usually starts in the 3rd month. Weight gain up to the 5th month is not usually very great. It could account for 25% of the total weight increase. The greatest increase occurs in the 5th, 6th and 7th months. However, it should not exceed 1 kilogram in any 1 week. Excessive weight gain at this time is associated with toxaemia and the doctor may ask you to watch your weight if she finds the weight gain excessive. After 7½ months the rate of weight increase slows down until the 9th month after which there is very often no weight gain in the last 4 weeks of pregnancy.

According to Dr Tom Brewer, an American obstetrician, nutrition is important. His theories are based on a series of controlled antenatal experiments, and go against the widely held belief that the baby is a parasite, and takes whatever it needs, regardless of the mother's nutrition.

He believes that even mild degrees of under-nutrition in the mother, especially in the last few weeks of pregnancy, can interfere with the normal growth and development of the baby's brain. He and his wife discuss this in their book, *What Every Pregnant Woman Should Know*, New York, 1979. Many doctors now feel that even 16 kg (35 pounds) and up is a reasonable weight gain for some women. In case of twins, 18 kg and above (40 to 50 pounds) weight gain may not be excessive.

DIET IN LABOUR

There is a widely held belief that if you have a glass of milk with clarified butter/ghee before going to the hospital, it helps. However, once labour is established (i.e. when one contraction lasts a whole minute), your digestion slows down greatly and the body concentrates on the birth.

At this stage of established labour, if you have eaten something heavy, it will remain in the stomach and make you feel like vomiting. On the other hand, light things eaten in labour will get digested and will have passed through the stomach, giving your body energy.

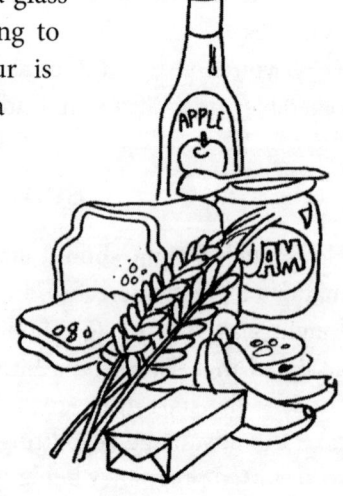

Therefore if you have started labour and are hungry, eat something light, high in carbohydrate. Do not eat anything with fat (butter/ghee), protein (non-vegetarian food/nuts/ dals/milk) or fibre (fruits/vegetables/dals).

You can have sips of water. If you feel you need some energy you could eat some sugar, glucose or honey. These things do not need time to get digested and get absorbed immediately by the body, giving you instant energy.

Mishri or rock sugar, sweets and lollipops, bananas, tetra-packed apple or lichi juice, plain boiled rice or boiled potatoes with salt can also be had.

Tea, coffee or fresh lime water/nimbupani should be avoided as they could cause acidity which can be a problem, if general anaesthesia has to be administered. Also avoid sour things like orange juice or tomato soup.

If your labour is well established, you will simply not have the desire to eat, even if your favourite dish is placed before you.

DIET WHEN BREASTFEEDING

Remember, when you are pregnant or when feeding the baby, you need a lot of nutrition; so it is a wrong time to diet. A woman who is feeding the baby needs more calories than a woman who is pregnant. In pregnancy, a woman needs 300 more calories than she normally would, whereas a woman feeding a baby would need 550 more calories.

Most women who feed their babies do feel ravenously hungry; a fact that shows you the importance of listening to your body and having faith in it. If you feel hungry, you must eat. A newborn baby needs about 120 calories per kilo per day, and weighs about 3 kilograms. Therefore the baby should get about 360 calories from milk. The mother uses more than 400 calories to nourish the baby.

In fact, a lot of weight that you put on during pregnancy consists of fat deposits, placed by nature, to be used up while feeding. If you continue to eat wisely, you can lose weight while feeding.

A woman feeding a baby should avoid too many spices, since these could give a peculiar smell to the milk, making it repulsive to the baby. She should drink plenty of fluids in any form, be it milk, soup, *nimbupani* or *lassi*, to make up for the loss of her body fluid in making breast milk. She does not need to drink lots of milk to make milk. In a relaxed mother the milk flows more easily. Less water does not reduce the amount of milk produced, but it makes the mother's urine very concentrated which is unhealthy for her.

A woman feeding a baby can have a normal non-spicy diet, with greater focus on pulses, green vegetables and milk.

Alcohol and cigarettes are to be avoided. But a glass of beer or wine is permissible as both have a very low alcohol content, which relaxes the mother. Beer, being barley-based, increases milk supply.

OUR TRADITIONAL RECIPES

A word about our traditional recipes of *laddoos, panjiri,* dry fruit or *mewa,* jaggery, or whatever else you may make, to feed a woman who has just delivered a baby. They contain ingredients that are traditionally believed to be beneficial to a woman who has just delivered a baby.

The point is to have the traditional recipes in moderation. Eat about 3 to 4 tablespoons of *panjiri,* or ½ or 1 *laddoo* with your early morning tea, when you know that activity will follow; or after a period of activity. Do not eat it as dessert after dinner and go to sleep. That is the best way to put on weight.

Overeating of anything heavy like ice-cream, chocolates, *mithai* or pastries can make you put on weight, so why blame *panjiri*?

An interesting example illustrating the wisdom of our traditional practices comes to mind. In parts of South India, a woman who has delivered a baby is given water to drink in which an iron rod has been boiled. This makes it a wonderful iron rich drink. On account of monthly periods and childbearing, women generally lack iron and therefore are often prescribed iron tablets. Boiled water would also be safer to drink, since boiling destroys germs or infection present in it.

TO GET THE MAXIMUM GOODNESS FROM YOUR FOOD

- Clear vegetable soup is very nutritious. All the vitamins, minerals, proteins, etc. from the vegetables are passed into the soup. Thick soups are not good, as flour and fat are used to thicken them.
- Greens, like kerae, palak, methi, sarson, bathua, cholai, should be washed first and then chopped. If you cut them first and then wash them, you will lose most of the water-soluble vitamins while washing.
- Keep your vegetables away from heat and light. Heat and bright sunlight destroy some of the vitamins. Further destruction comes with cooking, so that by the time you eat it, a fair amount of vitamins are lost. Boil potatoes whole.
- With fruits and vegetables avoid peeling if possible, or peel lightly, e.g. carrots, apples, pears. Wash vegetables and fruits before peeling, not afterward.
- Do not overcook vegetables; keep them crunchy. Try and cook just before eating, in order to avoid reheating. Avoid storing cooked vegetables in the fridge for more than 24 hours. When you reheat food, first leave it outside the fridge for about ½ an hour so that the change of temperature is not too sudden. Avoid overcooking vegetables to death. Steaming in the pressure cooker protects vitamins.
- It is best to use stainless steel utensils for cooking, since it is a metal that does not react to the food, like many other metals do. If you do not have them, the next best thing is to transfer food into stainless steel or plain glass bowls as soon as it is cooked.

POSITIONS IN LABOUR

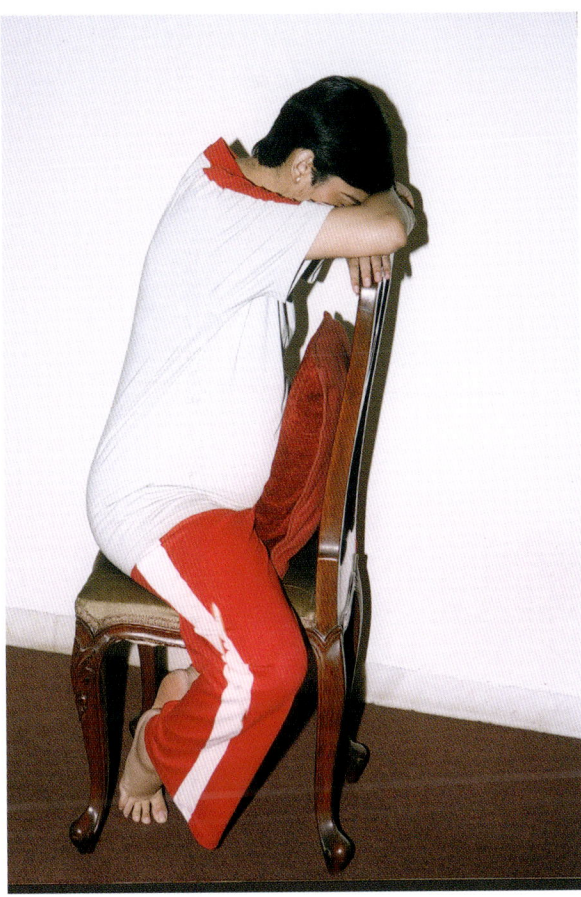

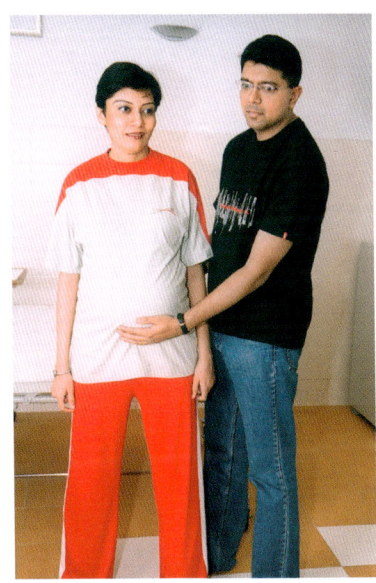

Stand facing the wall with your feet apart, bend forward and rest your head on your hands. Make sure that your back is straight and not arched.

To sit facing the back of a chair is a very comfortable position in labour. A cushion can be placed in front of the stomach for comfort. The knees should be below the hips.

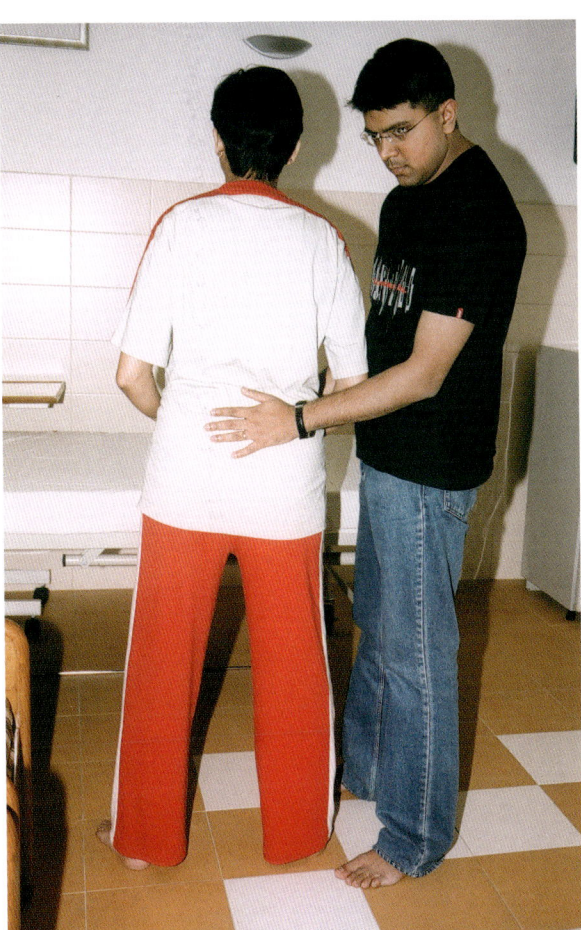

If your labour companion places one hand on your lower back and one on your lower abdomen when you have a contraction, it is comforting. (It can be done for you in whichever position you are.)

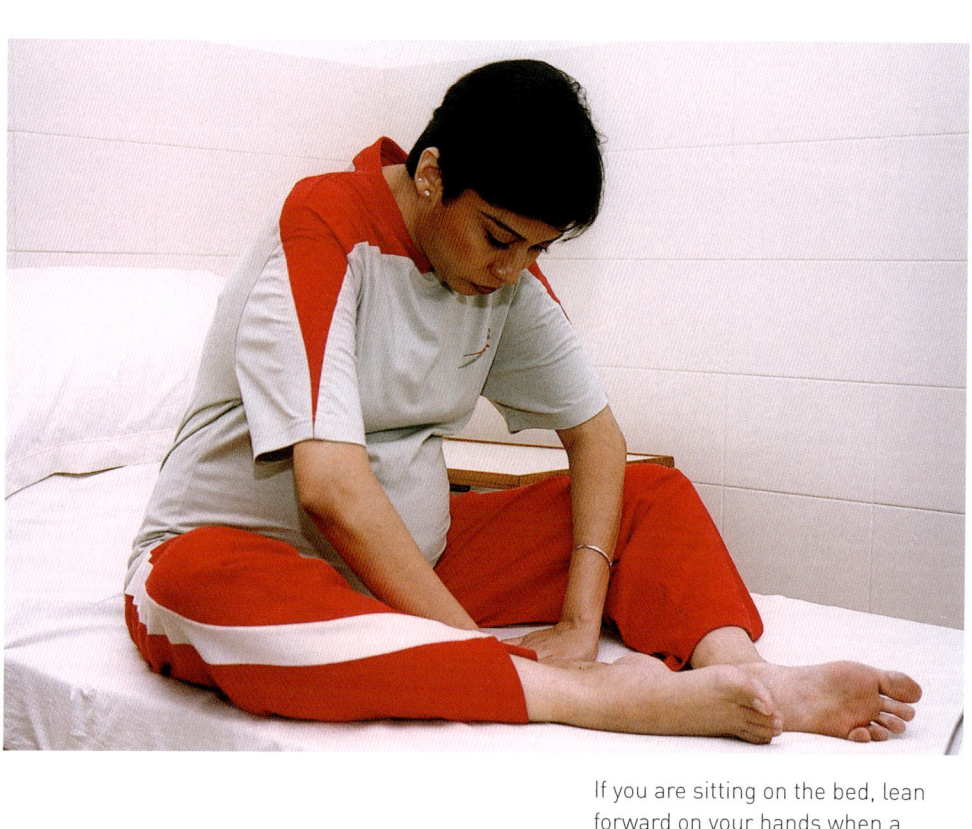

If you are sitting on the bed, lean forward on your hands when a contraction comes.

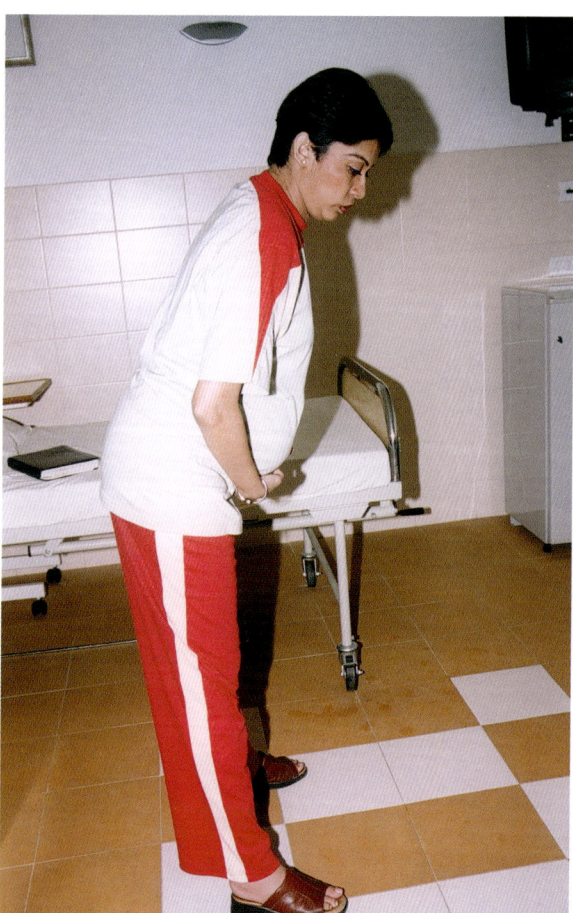

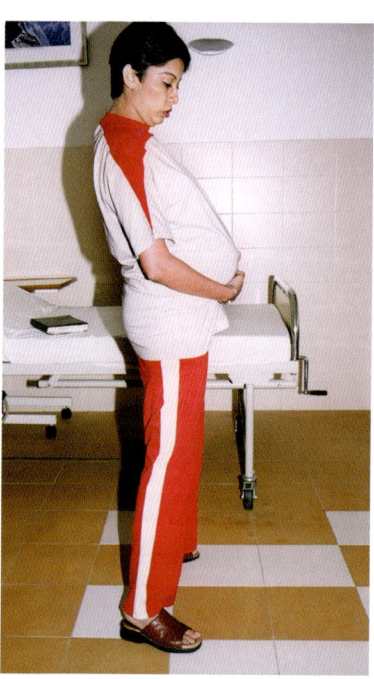

When walking in labour, stand, when a contraction comes, hold your abdomen, and circle with your hips.

POSITIONS IN LABOUR

BACKACHE IN LABOUR

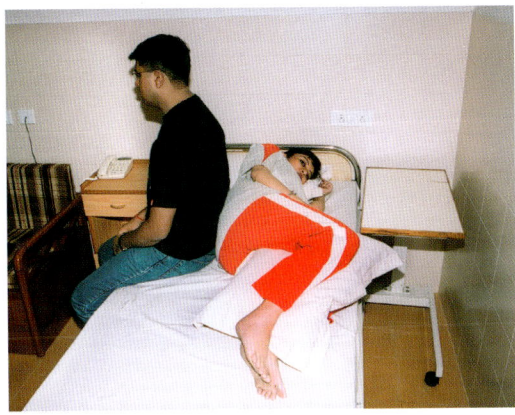

Your partner can sit back to back with you as you lie with a pillow between your legs.

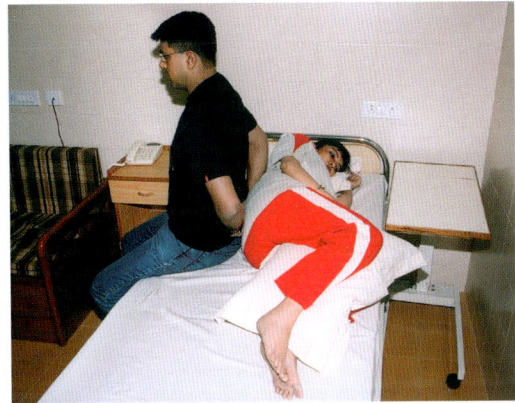

If you want greater pressure he can place his hands between his back and yours.

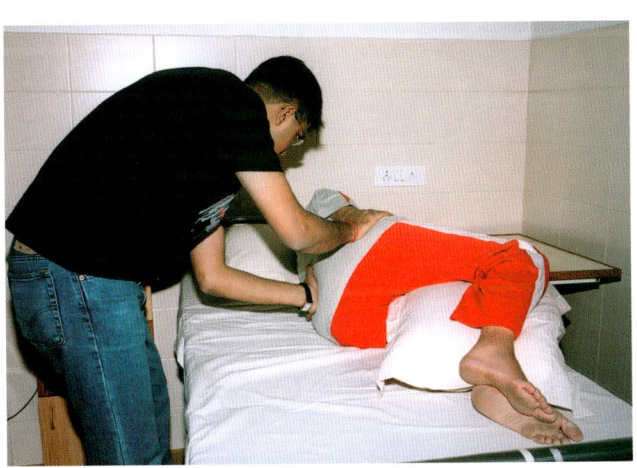

Or else he could massage your back with his palm as he holds your hip with the other hand to steady you.
He will find this easier to do if you shift towards the edge of the bed towards him so that he can rest the elbow of the hand with which he is massaging, on his abdomen or thigh.

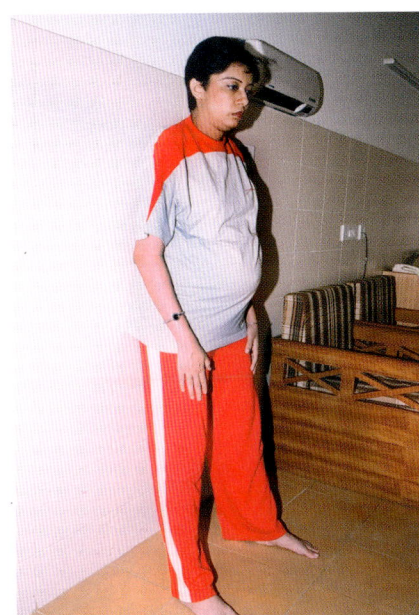

Standing with lower back pressed against the wall eases back pain in labour/during contractions.

POSITIONS IN LABOUR

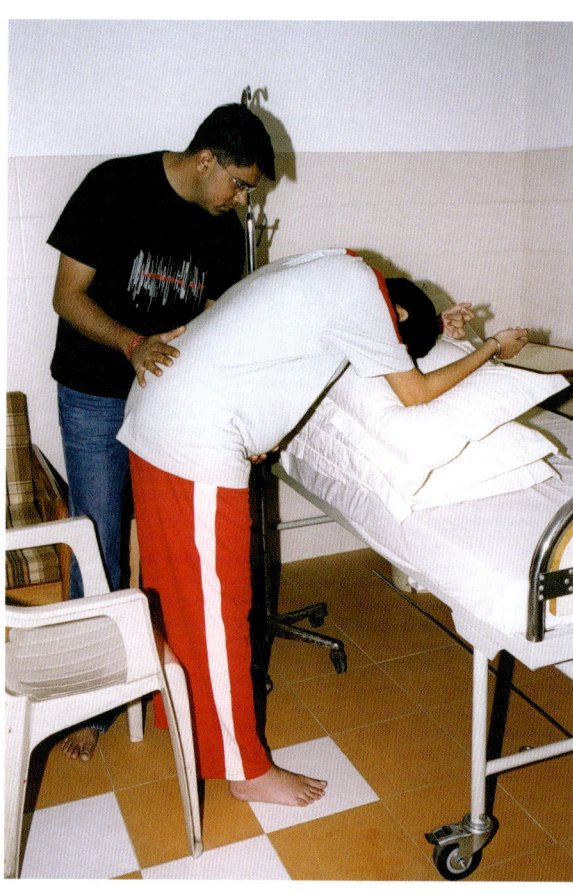

If you have the drip fixed on your hand or are too tired to walk, sit on a chair in front of the bed, and when the contraction comes, lean forward on a pile of pillows on the bed.

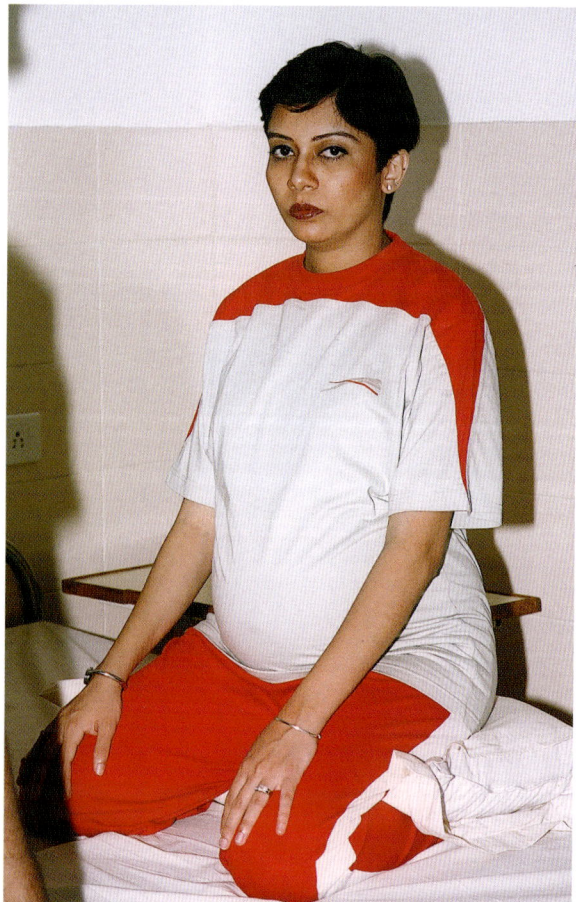

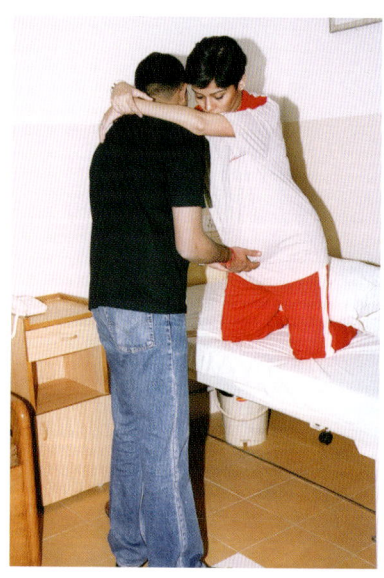

You could kneel on the bed with a pillow on the back of your legs, and when a contraction comes, get up and lean forward on your partner. Your partner could lightly stroke your lower abdomen as you do so.

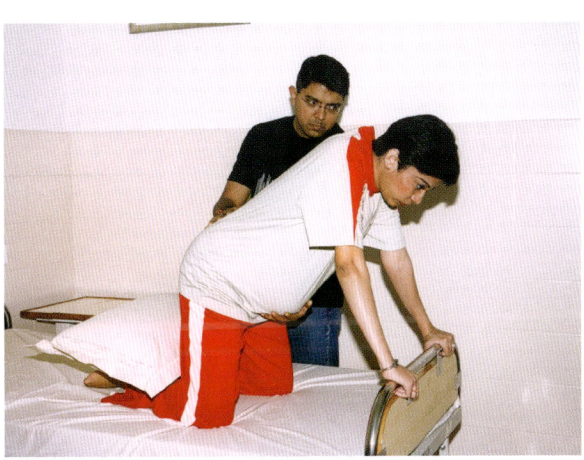

You could kneel on the bed with a pillow on the back of your legs, and when your contraction comes get up and lean forward to hold the headboard or footboard. If your partner is present he could place his palms on your lower abdomen and lower back.

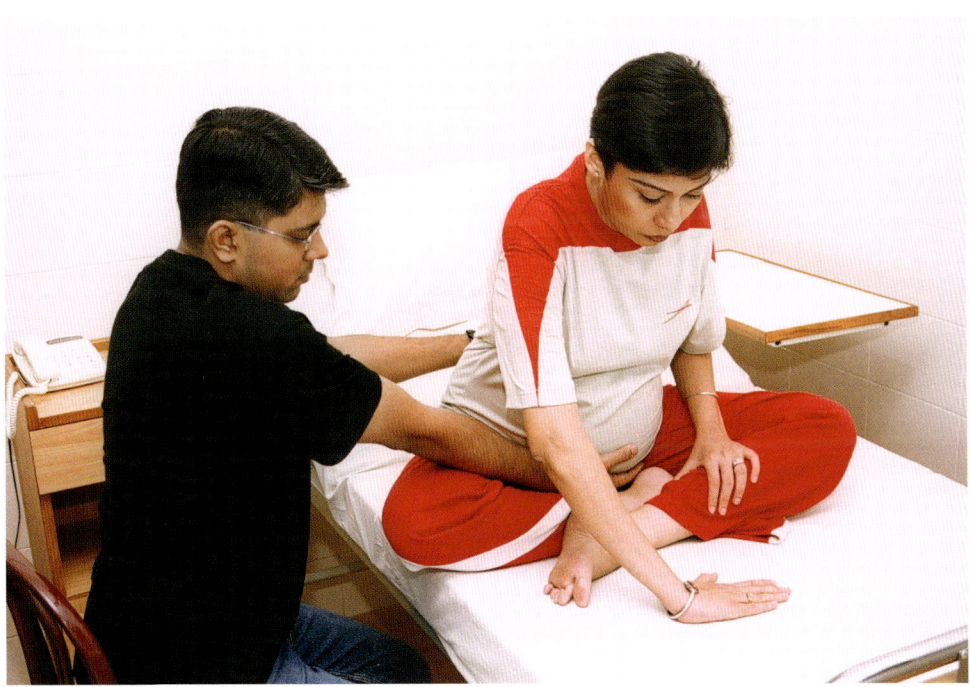

If you sit on the bed and lean forward when your contraction comes your labour partner can place his hands on your lower abdomen and lower back, as he sits by your bedside.

POSITIONS IN LABOUR

WHEN WATER BAG BURSTS

If your Water Bag Bursts in a gush of about one litre of water, some hours later you could start contractions. When contractions happen, you could leak water, in which case, the following positions could be used.

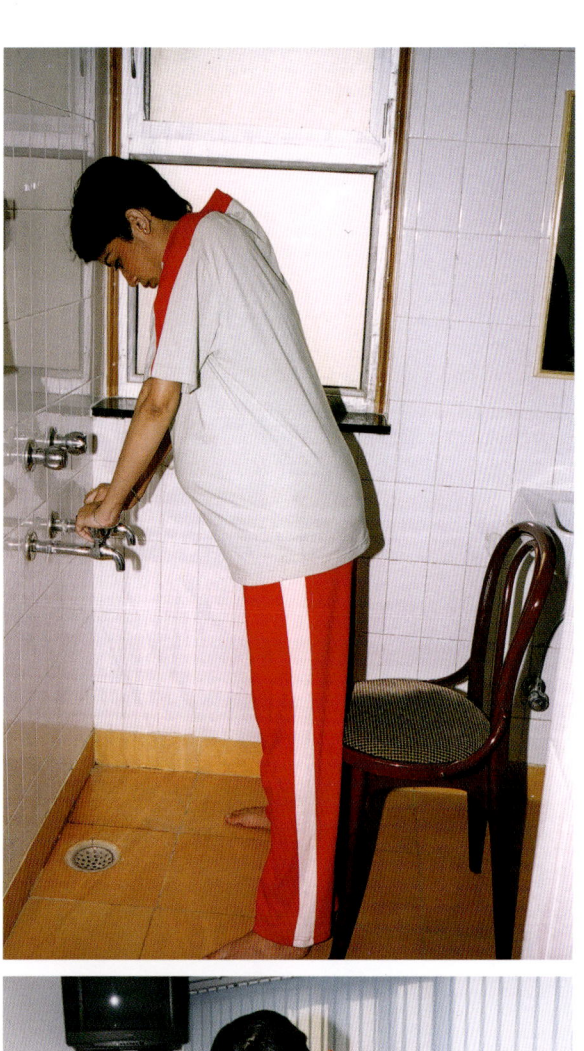

You could stand in the bathing area in the bathroom and lean forward holding the taps. The water that leaks could drain away.

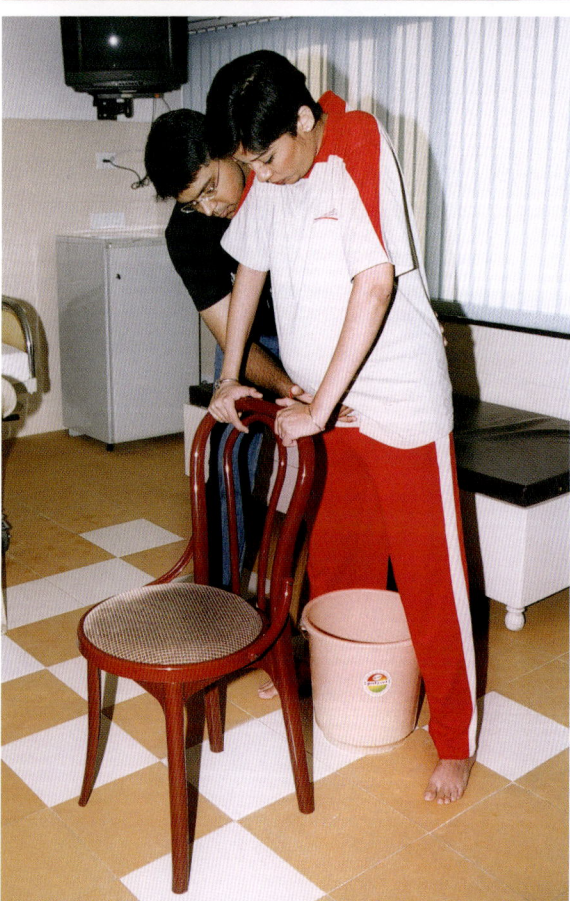

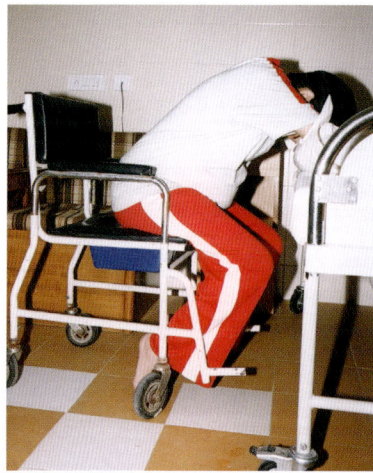

You could sit on a chair with a commode in front of the bed and lean forward on the bed when you have a contraction, the water will not wet you as it goes into the commode.

You could stand over a bucket, which could collect the drips, and stroll around the room when you don't have a contraction.

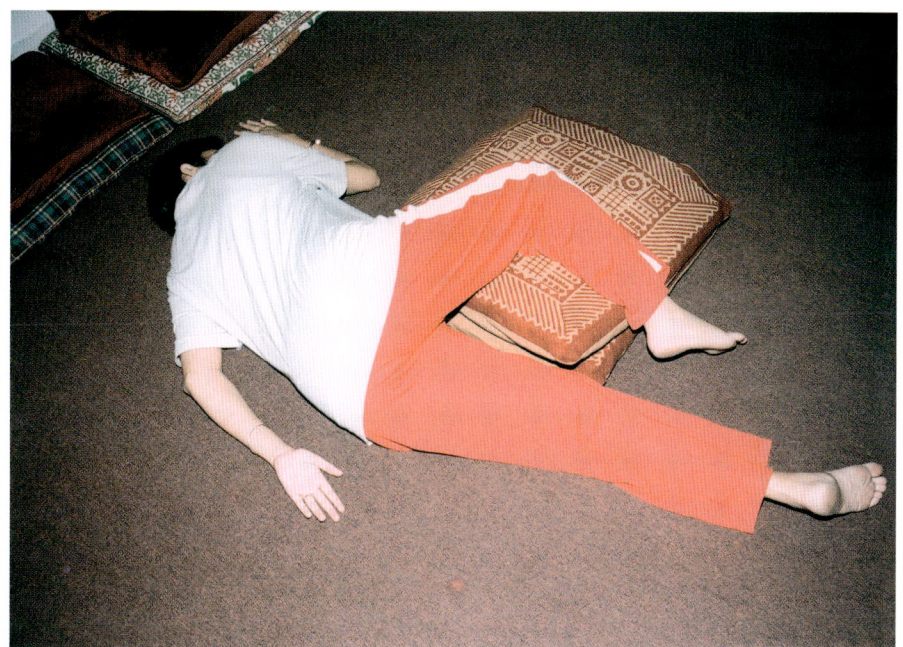

An excellent position for sleeping or relaxing, specially for those who have backache in pregnancy. Place a pile of cushions as high as your hips for resting your upper knee on, and place your lower arm alongside your backbone at the back. (see end of chapter, 'Some Simple Exercises')

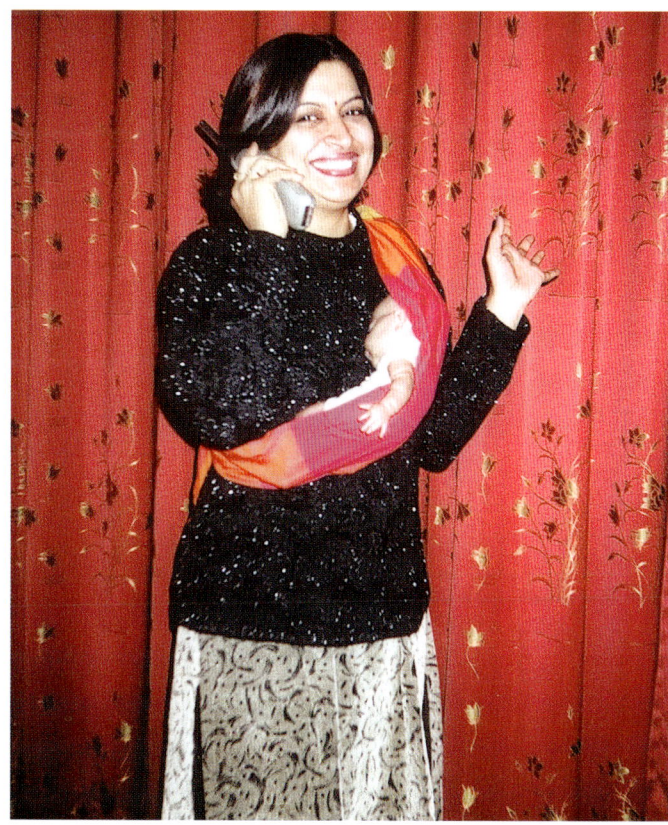

If you use a dupatta to make a sling for holding the baby, it leaves both your hands free. (see, 'A Sling For Baby' in chapter, 'After Childbirth')

DIET IN PREGNANCY

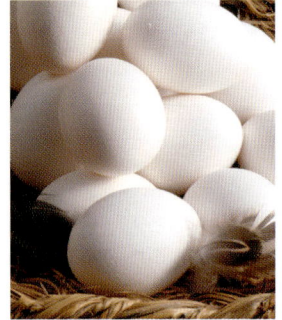
EGGS

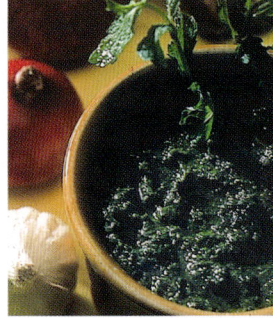
GREEN CHUTNEY

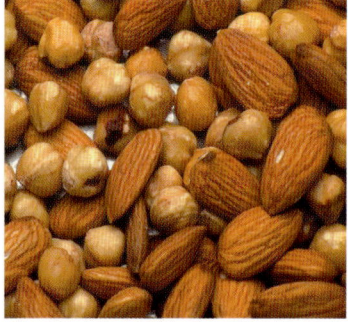
RAW NUTS AND ALMONDS

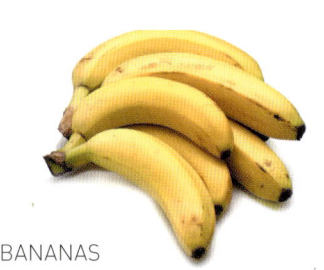
BANANAS

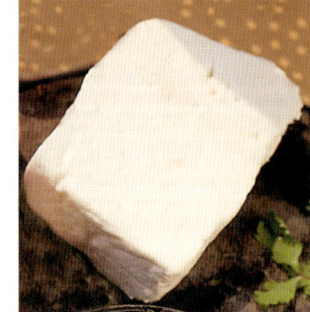
PANEER

CARROTS

KALA CHANNA SPROUTS

MILK

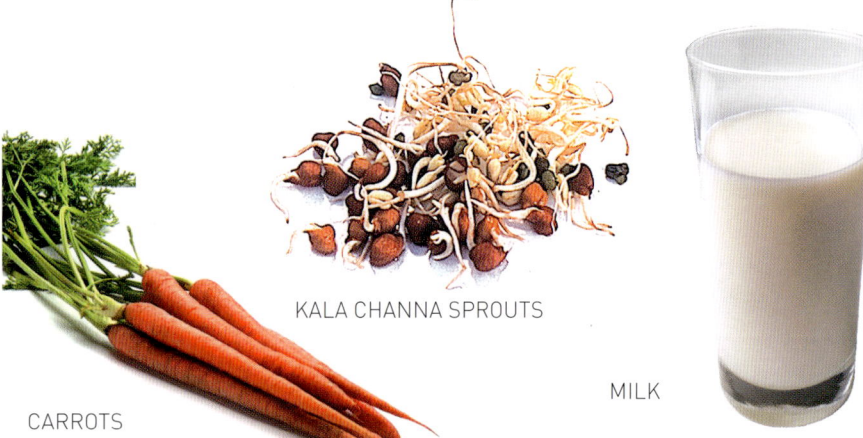

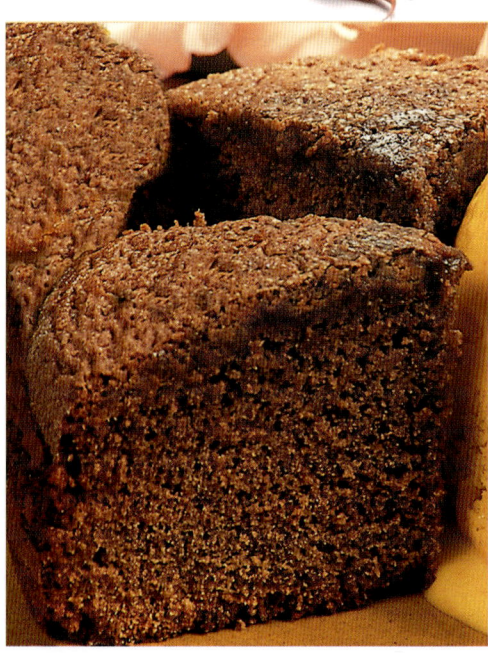

ATTA CAKE

Mix together:
2 cups atta
2 cups lal shakkar (gur sugar or grate gur & measure 2 cups)
½ tsp. Baking Powder
1½ tsp. Soda-bi-carb
1 tsp. Cinnamon (Dal chini) Powder

Then Add:
1 tsp. vanilla
⅔ cups oil or butter or ghee or margarine
¾ cup water

Mix together & add:
1 cup curd OR 3 eggs
Let the batter stand for a minimum of ½ hour before baking.
Bake as you would another cake in your oven.
(*Approximately 45 mins to 1 hour in gas oven*)

GHEE

If you take *ghee* regularly, but do not do much work in the house and do not go for regular walks either, it could result in extra weight and stiff joints, making delivery difficult. However, if you are active and if you are not overweight, and if you do not have any cholesterol problem, you can go ahead and have ghee.

Traditionally there is a belief that eating ghee in the ninth month helps to have an easy delivery. Research shows that ghee being a good fat, helps the perineum to plumps up and stretch easily.

Fats in the diet also help in the absorption of fat soluble vitamins A, D, E and K, during the process of digestion. Absorption of these vitamins would benefit the mother as per the table illustrated.

All these factors could be of significance in relation to childbirth. For instance, keeping infection away would be useful; strong bones and good skin could be of enormous help. Blood that clots could prevent haemorrhage (bleeding) post-birth, in mother and baby.

Also, in the ninth month, the baby gains maximum weight (200 gms per week) and the baby's brain is developing rapidly. The brain is made up of mostly fat and weight gain also requires fat. These may be the reasons behind this tradition.

1 gm of ghee has 9 calories. 1 tablespoon of ghee has 15 gm of ghee and therefore 135 calories. According to *Dietary Guidelines far Indians* published by the National Institute of Nutrition, Hyderabad, 1998, 'Visible fat intake should be increased during pregnancy and lactation to 30 grams and 45 grams respectively'.

15 gm of fat therefore falls within permissible limits. However, for today's aware, weight-conscious women, who do not want to put on too much weight, here are a couple of tips. When you add one tablespoon of ghee or butter to your diet in the 9th month, you can avoid other intake of calories like puddings, chocolates, cold drinks, foods with thick gravies, fried foods etc. Or you can increase your calorie expenditure by going for long walks, which will also be beneficial in preparing your body for an easy and natural childbirth.

One could have a tablespoon of pure homemade butter or a tablespoon of pure homemade ghee in the last month of pregnancy. Butter/ghee could be consumed with chappatis, parathas or dal, toast, etc.

TIPS ON WEIGHT CONTROL

RELAX
- Learn to relax before a party. When you are relaxed you will not have an urge to reach out for snacks. When you are jittery, you will tend to eat more. Things that can make you jittery are a lack of sleep and rest. Caffeine in coffee and colas can also make you jittery.

EAT REGULARLY
- Apart from the jitters, anxiety makes you overeat. When you

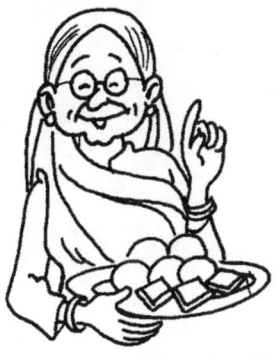

A RECIPE

YOU WILL NEED:

Ghee (clarified butter)	1 tbsp
Atta (whole wheat flour)/	
Sooji (cream of wheat)	1 tbsp
chhoti elaichi	
(small green cardamom)	1
Badam-(almonds)	2 to 3
Milk	1 glass
Sugar	to taste

METHOD:
Warm ghee, add sooji/atta to it and cook till light brown. Add milk and bring to a boil. Cook on a slow fire for 5 minutes so that the ghee blends with the milk. Add sugar, crushed elaichi and badam. Drink while hot the first thing in the morning starting from the 9th month and continuing till the birth. Some people have it post-birth, not pre-birth.

Source: Sonia Bajaj

Fat Soluble Vitamins	
Vitamin	Benefits
A	Prevents infection
D	Makes bones strong
E	Makes skin healthy
K	Helps in blood clotting

are anxious about some problem, you tend to find comfort in food. It is therefore important to eat at regular hours and not munch between meals. If you reach out for food every time you feel anxious, you will aggravate your weight problem and looking at your overweight self will lead you to further despair. It will give you a poor self-image and lack of confidence. You will tend to console yourself further with food, thus a vicious cycle will be formed.

TAKE RESPONSIBILITY

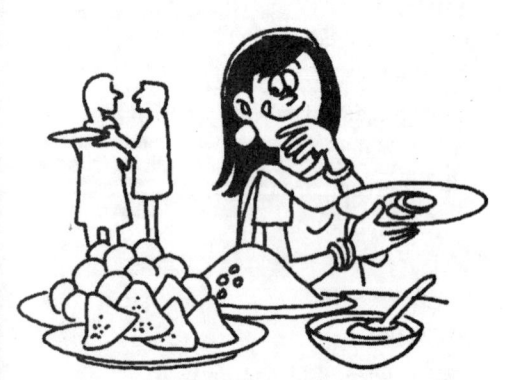

- If this applies to you, you should learn to take responsibility for your body and its needs. You should be in control of your food and not let your food control you. This does not mean that you should starve yourself for long periods and then overeat. If you do starve yourself, you are most likely to overeat, because when no food has been eaten, the blood sugar level drops and you crave food. Therefore it will not be surprising if you lose control. Never skip a meal. Regular eating habits protect you from hunger pangs that make you reach out for the wrong foods. More important, regular food intake makes the body function more efficiently.

AVOID TEMPTATION

- Do not go where you know you will find temptation. At weddings and parties, do not stand near the table laden with fattening food.

LIMIT YOUR PORTIONS

- At home, serve yourself in a *thali* and eat, rather than dipping into dishes just to taste, or just to finish that litttle bit of rice or *chappati or* to give others company, or
- to finish left-overs, to finish a dish full of expensive ingredients, or to clean up your child's plate—the list is endless.

EAT SLOWLY

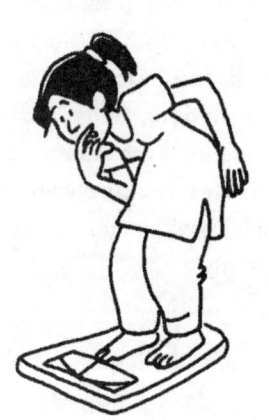

- Take at least 20 minutes over your meal. It takes about that much time for the stomach to tell the brain it is no longer hungry. Chew slowly, at least 20 times and savour each mouthful. It will give you greater satisfaction from your food.

WEIGH YOURSELF REGULARLY

- Weigh yourself on the same weighing scale once a week. Don't fool yourself that a few kilos here or there is not much. Think of the stuff you buy in the market. 5 kilos is a lot of weight.

MAKE SILENT EFFORTS

- Do not talk about your efforts to change your food habits, as people will try and talk you out of it. If you are a compulsive eater, keep the right kind of snacks around; moong sprouts, boiled potatoes, carrots, cucumber, seasonal fruits, chana.

WATER, NOT BEVERAGES
- Learn to drink plain, clean sparkling water instead of tea, coffee, sherbets, colas, etc. Set yourself a goal as to what weight you want to achieve. Then work towards it steadily.

DISCOURAGE FOOD GIFTS
- Do not encourage people to pamper you with food.

DO NOT DIET
- There is an interesting book called *Dieting Makes You Fat* (London, 1984) by Geoffrey Cannon. The author has spent years of his life following various diet plans. According to him, frequent dieting gives the body starvation signals, and when food is once again available the body reacts by overstoring, being unable to differentiate between a weight loss regime and serious food deprivation. He further says that the rate of the breakdown of food is considerably reduced while dieting, as this is one of the survival tactics the body uses when food is scarce. This sluggish metabolism makes weight loss more difficult.

INDULGE OCCASIONALLY
- Constant yet moderate eating habits, with occasional indulgence on weekends, is the best path to try and follow.

CONSULT A PROFESSIONAL
- It is a good idea to consult an expert on nutrition to chalk out a diet for you in accordance with your taste and preferences. Nutrition experts can be found in home science colleges, hospitals and nursing homes and in weight reduction clinics. They take into account your lifestyle. Do you cook and do other housework or are you physically inactive? They will consider whether you are pregnant, feeding the baby, or are just a simple housewife. Are you a vegetarian or a non-vegetarian? Taking all these factors into account, a diet chart will be made up specially for you.
- And lastly, if you are putting on weight in leaps and bounds, although you are not eating much, get yourself checked by a doctor for any physical problem like malfunction of the thyroid gland.

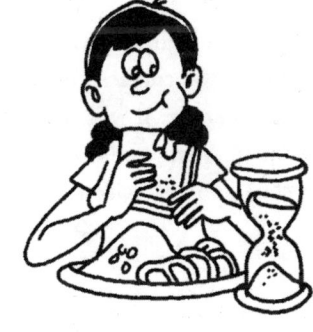

6

SOME SIMPLE EXERCISES

During pregnancy, exercises should be done keeping in mind the changes that happen in a woman when she is pregnant. For instance, her muscles and joints get relaxed. This causes changes and strain in certain parts of her body. Any exercise regime must take this into consideration. The following exercises are specifically designed for the physical and emotional changes a pregnant woman experiences.

GROUNDING

This exercise will help you sit up straight in the correct posture to do your exercise. It will also calm you and quieten your mind before you start your exercise regimen.

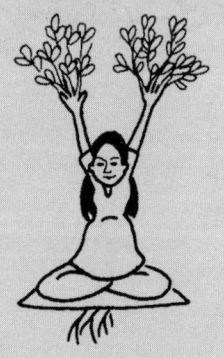

STEP 1
Sit cross-legged on a firm surface, be it a carpet / *dari* / yoga mat / firm bed surface. As you sit cross-legged, become aware of the areas of your body that are touching the ground.

STEP 2
Now imagine that you are a plant, and from the areas of your body that are touching the ground, imagine that there are roots growing down into the ground. Your backbone is like a stem that rises straight and strong out of the ground. Your head on the top is like a flower on the top of the stem and it reaches up towards the sun. Feel the top of your head reach up without raising your chin.

STEP 3
Breathe in slowly and deeply the nourishment from the roots straight up to your head and slowly exhale. Imagine you are exhaling all your tension with your breath. As you breathe in imagine that you are drawing nourishment from the roots straight up to your head.

Do this for 2 minutes.

NECK EXERCISE

In order to mobilize and strengthen the neck and shoulder muscles, the following exercises are helpful. It also helps relieve tension in the neck and shoulder muscles.

STEP 1: Sit cross-legged with the back straight. Keep the head and the neck in one straight line.
STEP 2: Incline the head slightly downwards, so that the chin moves towards the chest.

STEP 3: Then straighten the head again and take it backwards with your mouth open, so that you are looking at the ceiling. Close your mouth, feeling the stretch in front of the neck and hold the position for a count of 6.
STEP 4: Bring the head back to starting position.
Do this 3 times.

SHOULDER ROTATION

Good for the upper back. This exercise helps relieve pain in the upper back and nape of the neck.

STEP 1: Sit cross-legged with the back straight. Keep the head and neck in a straight line.
STEP 2: Bring shoulders forward.
STEP 3: Raise shoulders up to your ears.
STEP 4: Thrust shoulders backwards, so that chest juts outwards.
STEP 5: Bring shoulders back to starting position.
STEP 6: Repeat these movements in one fluid motion, so that you make a circle with your shoulders.
STEP 7: Make circles in the opposite direction. Do 5 circles in each direction.

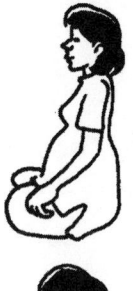
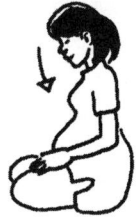
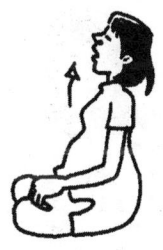

DEEP BREATHING

This is not a simple exercise. You are exercising all the muscles of your carriage. It provides a lot of oxygen to you and your baby. Besides, when you breathe in, the diaphragm presses on the abdominal organs, massaging and invigorating them.

POSITION

Sit cross-legged with the back straight. Keep the head and neck in a straight line.

STEP 1: Take a short breath in, then exhale slowly through pursed lips, to the maximum.
STEP 2: Let your lungs naturally fill up with air when exhalation is complete.
STEP 3: Breathe normally for about 3 breaths.
STEP 4: Repeat the first 3 steps.
Do this 3 times.
It is best to do this exercise early in the morning near plants (since, when the sun shines, plants make oxygen). Moreover, exposure to the morning sun makes Vitamin D which helps in calcium absorption. There is also less dust and vehicle exhaust in the atmosphere at that time.

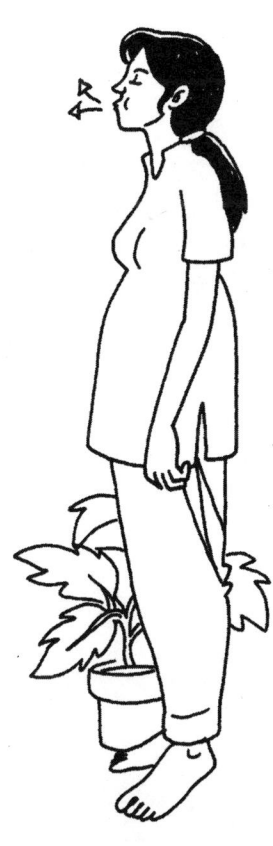

BUST EXERCISE

This exercise exercises the pectoral muscles, which are muscles of the chest. The pectorals hold the breasts in place. The breasts themselves are made up of specialized tissue that produces milk (glandular tissue) as well as fatty tissue.

This exercise strengthens the pectoral muscles and helps lift and firm the breasts.

SECTION A

STEP 1: Sit cross-legged with the back straight and your head and neck in a straight line.
STEP 2: Join both palms together under the breasts in a horizontal position, that is, with the fingertips pointing straight ahead.
STEP 3: Press the palms firmly together and hold to a count of 10.
STEP 4: Release pressure on both palms.
STEP 5: Repeat 3 times.

SECTION B

STEP 1: Now join both palms together in front of the breasts, in a slanting position.
STEP 2: Press the palms firmly together and hold to a count of 10.
STEP 3: Release pressure on both the palms.
STEP 4: Repeat 3 times.

SECTION C

STEP 1: Join both palms together with the fingertips pointing to your chin.
STEP 2: Press palms firmly together and hold to a count of 10.
STEP 3: Release pressure on both palms.
STEP 4: Repeat this 3 times.

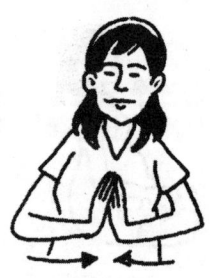

Note: The palms are joined together as when greeting someone with a 'Namaste'.
When doing the exercise the palms should not touch your body or rest on your body.
The central position of the exercise (SECTION B), with palms joined in a slant in front of the breasts, is to be done when breastfeeding, for 6 months after the birth of the baby.

PELVIC FLOOR EXERCISE

The pelvic floor muscles support the womb. They help to hold the extra weight of the growing uterus in pregnancy. Exercising these muscles helps to strengthen them and maintains their shape.

POSITION

Sit cross-legged. Can also be done while standing or lying down. Start with Exercise A. After 3 days start Exercise B. After 3 more days graduate to Exercise C.

Exercise A
STEP 1: Exhale. Leave your pelvic floor absolutely relaxed, as when passing urine.

STEP 2: Now imagine that you interrupt or stop the flow of urine for a while, by a slight contraction of the muscles.
STEP 3: Repeat the above steps 3 times.

Exercise B
STEP 1: Exhale. Relax the pelvic floor.
STEP 2: Imagine that you want to pass urine badly, but you are at a public toilet and have to wait in the queue; and as you wait, you have to control the passing of urine by a strong contraction of your muscles.
STEP 3: Hold the contraction for a count of 6 and release. Exhale and repeat the contraction twice. Your anus might also contract slightly, that does not matter, since your anus, vagina, and urethra are in one band of muscles. You might feel a slight tightening above the pubic hairline. You should not feel a tightening around the navel of your abdomen. If you do, it is a sign that you should locate the contraction backwards towards the anus instead. You are now ready for the final step of the exercise.

Exercise C
STEP 1: Exhale.
STEP 2: Contract your pelvic floor muscles a little bit. Count to 6.
STEP 3: Contract your pelvic floor muscles a little more. Count to 6.
STEP 4: Contract your pelvic floor muscles the maximum you can. Count to 6.
STEP 5: Exhale slowly and gently release or let go of your pelvic floor muscles, while you exhale.
STEP 6: Breathe normally for 2 breaths, and repeat.

Repeat this exercise 5 times, taking two normal breaths in between, each time.

If you develop an ache in the muscles, it is because these muscles are not used to being exercised. The pain is like the pain you would get in your arm if you played badminton after many days. So do not stop the exercise, but do it in one continuous contraction to the count of 6, instead.

Repeat at least 5 times.

ANKLE MOVEMENTS

This exercise has its base in yoga. It exercises the ankles, a part of the body not generally exercised. It feels good, since the strain of the extra weight of pregnancy is carried by this area of the body.

STEP 1: Sit with one leg outstretched, the other leg bent at the knee, and the lower part of the bent leg (just above the ankle) resting on the thigh of the outstretched leg. Rest your back against the wall if you like.
STEP 2: Hold the bent leg just above the ankle with one hand; and with the other hand rotate the foot from the ankle.
STEP 3: Rotate the foot 5 times clockwise and 5 times anti-clockwise. Repeat with the other leg.

AN EXERCISE FOR EVERY WOMAN

Women need to do this exercise always. Beginning in pregnancy, for the rest of their lives.
Done mildly for 40 days after delivery (Exercise B), it promotes healing. Thereafter do Exercise C. It helps regain the pre-pregnant tightness of these muscles.
At approximately 50 years of age, when a woman exercises her pelvic floor muscles they remain strong and support the uterus.
If they sag and lose their ability to support the uterus, an operation may be performed for a prolapsed uterus.
It is also to be done by a woman who has never been pregnant, and by women who have had a caesarean section. Lifting something heavy and age can also slacken these muscles.

PRECAUTIONS

Always exhale before starting this exercise.

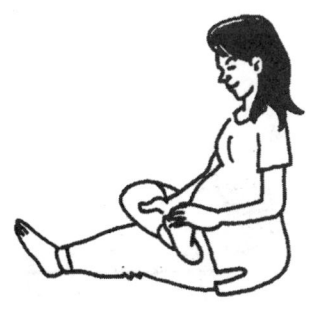

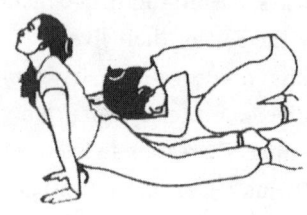

FORWARD BACKWARD

This exercise provides relief from general back pain and sciatica pain in pregnancy.

1. Sit on your heels with knees bent.
2. Separate your knees.
3. Bend forward, place forehead on the floor and place your palms in front of you on the floor.
4. Stretch palms forward at arm's length and rise on your knees.
5. Separate your feet, placing them in line with your knees.
6. Lunge forward to look up at the ceiling and lower your pelvic area towards the floor.
7. Hold for a count of 6 or 10 and then return to starting position.

Repeat 3 to 5 times

PELVIC LIFT

Strengthens the back muscles and relieves lower backache or feeling of congestion in the groin.

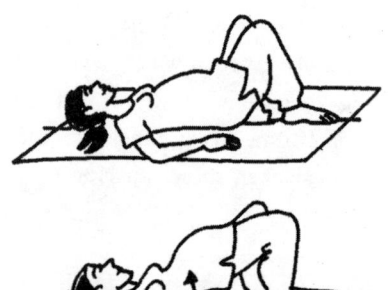

STEP 1: Lie down flat on your back. Bend both legs at knees and place feet on the floor.
STEP 2: Now put your weight on both feet and raise your hips off the floor.
STEP 3: Once raised, stay in position for at least 10 counts.
STEP 4: Then gently lower yourself back to the floor.

Do once or twice. Help in lifting the pelvis may be taken from someone if you are unable to do so independently. Someone can stand by your side next to your hips and place both arms around your lower back and help you rise off the floor.

KNEE-CHEST POSITION

When you are upright all day, the organs hang from the spine as a flag hangs from a pole. When you position yourself for this exercise by going on all fours, the organs hang from the spine like clothes from a line. Hence this exercise relaxes the back.

When you do this exercise, the weight of the pregnant uterus is shifted away from the pelvic floor and the spine. It therefore takes care of backache and radiating pains in the hips and legs.

This exercise also feels good if you have a gastric problem and are wanting to burp to relieve yourself.

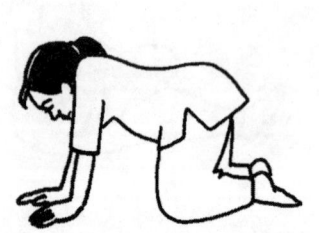

STEP 1: Kneel on the floor with knees slightly apart.
Then go forward on all fours, by placing your palms on the floor in front of you directly under your shoulder joints. Keep your head down and back straight.

Keep your head down all the while. Raising the head will tend to encourage the hollowing or caving in of the back. If the back is allowed to hollow, it can give rise to a backache.

Stay for a while in this position.

STEP 2: Go down/putting your elbows in place of your palms, and point palms towards opposite elbows.

STEP 3: Rest your head on your arms. If your stomach pushes against the thighs, separate your knees farther, so that your stomach fits in the hollow between your thighs. Secondly, guard against hollowing of the back. If hollowing occurs, correct it by gently pulling in your stomach.

STEP 4: Stay in position as long as you comfortably can. Breathe normally. While in position you will feel a rush of blood towards the face which will make your face warm. Do not worry.

This exercise is to be done once. The longer the position is maintained, the greater the benefit derived from it.

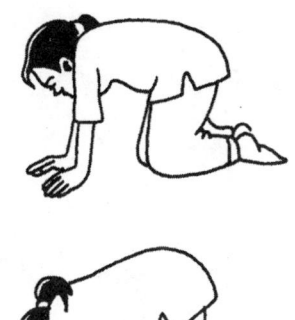

PRECAUTION

If you have high blood pressure, only do Step 1 of this exercise, i.e. stay in the all-fours position, avoid getting the head down.

LEG LIFT

In pregnancy there is a tendency to form varicose veins in the legs. Varicose veins are dark-looking veins that appear above or below the knees as a result of pooling of impure blood in the legs. Due to the congestion in the groin region impure blood cannot easily flow back to the heart for purification. This exercise helps prevent varicose veins by assisting the blood to flow back towards the heart past the groin area. It soothes the legs.

STEP 1: Lie on your side with one arm stretched outwards under your head, and the palm of the other arm placed in front of you. Place a pillow between your abdomen and the floor.

STEP 2: Raise the upper leg higher than your hip.

STEP 3: Hold for a count of 6.

STEP 4: Gently come back to the starting position. Repeat 3 to 4 times with each leg.

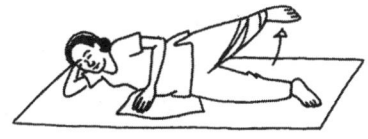

PRECAUTIONS

If you are prone to leg cramps, do not point your toe as you raise the leg. It will give you a cramp.

CURLING LEAF

Takes strain off the back while you are getting up and reduces the possibility of backache.

STEP 1: Lie flat on your back. Bend the left leg at the knee, placing the foot next to the knee of the outstretched leg. Stretch the right arm behind your head.

STEP 2: Put the weight of your body on the foot of the bent left leg.

STEP 3: Roll your body in the opposite direction, that is, to the right.

STEP 4: Simultaneously, as you roll on to the right side, bring your left palm to rest on the floor, in front of your abdomen.

STEP 5: Now straighten your left leg and rise up with your weight supported by your elbows and your palms.

Repeat with the other leg.

Practise 4 times till perfected. Then use simply as a way of getting up.

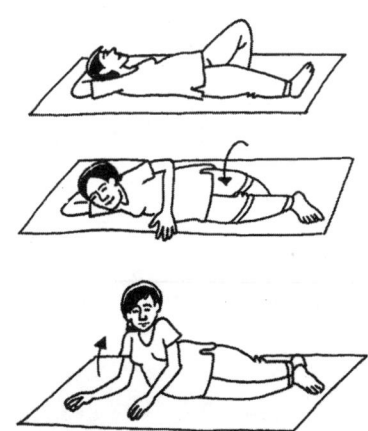

LEG SWING

There are 3 joints in the pelvis which spread slightly apart during delivery.

The present-day lifestyle of sitting on chairs all the time makes these joints inflexible. This exercise is to make them flexible, by bringing some movement in them.

POSITION
Stand with your hands on your hips and feet placed normally.

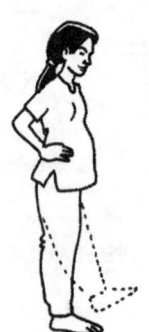

Exercise A
STEP 1: Tilt very slightly to the left side and swing the right leg forward and then backward 4 times.
STEP 2: Repeat with the other leg.

The swing forward and backward should not be exaggerated. About 1 foot forward and 1 foot backward is fine. Done overenthusiastically, it could cause an ache in the sacroiliac joints that have already been softened by hormones in preparation for birth.

You tend to lose balance, therefore pause, at the starting position between each forward and backward swing.

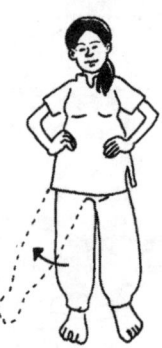

Exercise B
STEP 1: Stand with hands on hips.
STEP 2: Swing one leg sideways and out, then bring back to the starting position. Repeat 3 times.
STEP 3: Repeat with the other leg.

PELVIC TILTING

This exercise relieves lower backache and also helps retain abdominal tone, so that after your baby is born, the abdomen will tone up faster and more easily.

Your bony pelvic basin houses your reproductive organs like your ovaries and uterus. As the uterus balloons up with pregnancy, it spills out of the pelvic basin, putting its weight on the abdominal wall. The baby lies on the abdominal wall as though it were lying in a hammock. This weight on the abdominal wall puts pressure on the lower back muscles which begin to ache. It also causes the abdominal wall to stretch to its maximum and lose its tone and elasticity, giving rise to stretch marks.

This exercise tilts the pelvis in a way that the contents of the pelvis that press the abdominal wall are pushed inwards, so that their weight is taken by the bony pelvis during the duration of the exercise. This gives respite to the abdominal wall from stretching and relieves backache.

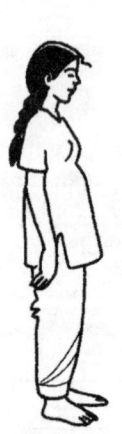

Exercise A
STEP 1: Stand normally.
STEP 2: Exhale.
STEP 3: Bend slightly at the knees.
STEP 4: Tilt your pubic hair area towards your navel, and slouch your

shoulders forward, so that the hollow of your back straightens out.
STEP 5: Hold the position for a count of 6.
STEP 6: Release and go back to the starting position
Repeat 5 times.

Exercise B
If you are fairly advanced in pregnancy you could do this exercise in a lying down position.

STEP 1: Lie down flat on your back. Bend legs at the knees and place feet flat on the floor.
STEP 2: Place a folded hand towel or napkin in the hollow of your back.
STEP 3: Exhale.
STEP 4: Tighten the buttock muscles and draw in the lower abdomen.
STEP 5: Simultaneously flatten the hollow of your back against the floor and press on the folded towel.
STEP 6: Hold for a count of 6.
STEP 7: Release, breathe normally twice, then repeat.
Repeat 5 times.

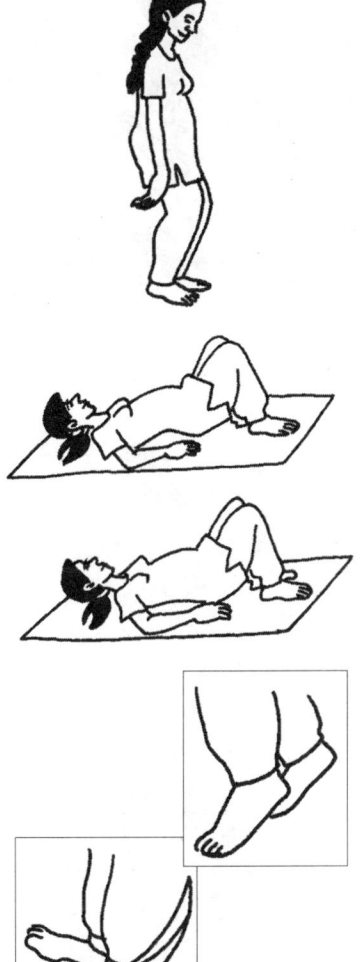

WALKING FOR CRAMPS AND ARCHES OF THE FOOT

Cramps can sometimes occur due to lack of blood circulation. This exercise gives a boost to blood circulation in your lower limbs.

STEP 1: Stand normally. You should have about 6 feet of open space for walking.
STEP 2: Walk across the 6-foot space on your toes.
STEP 3: Then walk back on your heels.
STEP 4: Finally walk on the outer sides of your feet.
Do once every day before bedtime. Sometimes cramps can also occur due to lack of calcium, magnesium, Vitamin B or E. If cramps do not get alleviated with walking, check your diet.

SQUATTING

While squatting, the pelvic inlet, outlet, and canal are at their widest. Those using the squatting type toilet are at an advantage as it exercises your joints and muscles without having to do much. Use it more frequently if you have one in the house.

Squatting correctly positions the growing baby and the uterus. It also cures constipation.

STEP 1: Squat as when using an Indian toilet. If you are well advanced in pregnancy, with a big stomach, follow these steps:
STEP 2: Stand normally, with your bottom touching the wall.
STEP 3: Now rise on your toes.
STEP 4: Go down into a squat.

PRECAUTION

Squatting should not be done by a woman who has had a stitch put on the mouth of the uterus by the doctor, nor by one who is bleeding in pregnancy, or who is on bed rest because of a low-lying placenta.
Squatting should also be avoided in case of severe or painful varicose veins or piles.

SOME SIMPLE EXERCISES

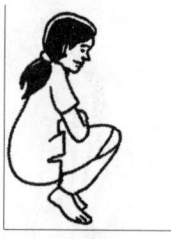
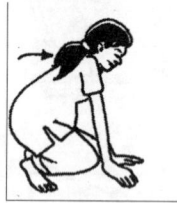
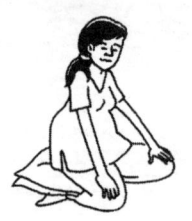

STEP 5: Do not go into a complete squat, remain in a slightly raised position.
STEP 6: Rest your lower back against the wall, and spread your knees as wide apart as you can.
STEP 7: Stay for at least 2 minutes in the final position.
STEP 8: Now go forward on your hands and then your knees to come out of the squatting position.

In the 9th month when the baby is in a head-down position, in order to encourage the fixing or the engagement of the baby's head, instead of squatting, one could sit with knees bent and a couple of cushions on one's calves.

This position would cause the pelvic structure to be raised to above the level of the knees, with a forward tilt to it, so that the angle becomes perfect for the baby to enter the pelvic inlet. This position, called 'Optimal Foetal Positioning', was advocated by Jean Sutton and Pauline Scott, midwife and childbirth educator, respectively, from New Zealand. It can be adopted by a woman as she watches TV or when she is sitting on the bed.

AUM BREATHING

This exercise has its base in yoga and is relaxing both for the mother and the baby. (Source: Swami Satyanand, Bihar School of Yoga)

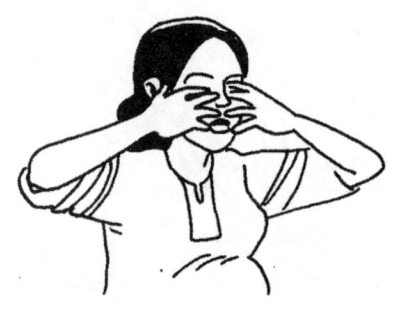

STEP 1: Sit cross-legged with the back straight. Keep the head and neck in a straight line. Place your thumbs firmly on the small triangular flap before the ear orifice. In this way you will block out any distraction caused by surrounding sounds.
Place the 2 fingers after your thumb lightly on your eyes.
Place the next 2 fingers, one above and one below the lips.
STEP 2: Breathe in.
STEP 3: As you breathe out or exhale say the word *Aum*.
Repeat 5 times without a break. If, while doing this exercise you feel breathless, take a pause by taking a sigh, that is, a deep inhalation and exhalation, in between the *Aum* breaths.

RELAXATION

It is very important for a woman to remain as relaxed as she can through pregnancy. A good time to practise relaxation is when you know you are not going to need to rush off in 10 minutes, when all your work is done, when you do not expect to be called or made to answer the telephone or doorbell.

Lie down quietly and allow your mind and body 5 to 10 minutes to quieten down. Use this time to also shift around and find a comfortable position to relax in, taking cushions, pillows, sheets or blankets as required. Once settled, allow your thoughts to pour in. Close your eyes and watch your thoughts in a detached way, as though you are watching a movie on the screen. Be detached: do not judge your thoughts; simply watch them for about 10 to 15 minutes.

Now try to do some conscious relaxation. Tape the following relaxation and play it to yourself or have someone read it to you:

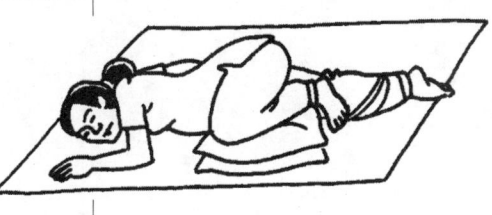

Relax the toes, feet and ankles.
Relax the nerves that hold the muscles of my toes, feet and ankles.
Relax my calves.
Relax the nerves that hold the muscles of my calves.
Relax my knees.
Relax the nerves that hold the muscles of my knees.
Relax my thighs.
Relax the nerves that hold the muscles of my thighs.
Now my lower limbs are relaxed and will not get unrelaxed.
Relax my pelvic floor.
Relax the nerves that hold the muscles of my pelvic floor.
Relax my buttocks.
Relax the nerves that hold the muscles of my buttocks.
Relax my womb and my lower abdomen.
Relax the nerves that hold the muscles of my lower abdomen.
Now my lower abdomen is relaxed and will not get unrelaxed.
Relax my back.
Relax my shoulder blades.
Relax the nerves that hold the muscles of my back.
Now my back is relaxed and will not get unrelaxed.
Relax my upper arms.
Relax my lower arms.
Relax my palms and fingers.
Relax the nerves that hold the muscles of my arms.
Now my arms are relaxed and will not get unrelaxed.
Relax my neck.
Relax the nerves that hold the muscles of my neck.
Now my neck is relaxed and will not get unrelaxed.
Relax my chin and face.
Relax the nerves that hold the muscles of my chin and face.
Now my face is relaxed and will not get unrelaxed.
Relax the top of my head.
Relax the back of my head.
Relax the nerves that hold the muscles of my head.
Now my head is relaxed and will not get unrelaxed.
Now relaxation is seeping into my brain.
Relax the nerves that hold the muscles of my brain.
Now my brain is relaxed and will not get unrelaxed.

Keep lying down with your eyes closed.
After relaxation do not get up suddenly. First become aware of your surroundings. Remember the room in which you are lying, and the furniture/doors/windows in it. Slowly move your hands and feet. Rise gently.

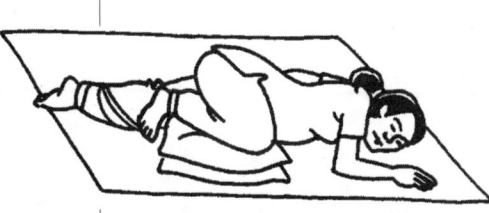

SOME SIMPLE EXERCISES

A Prayer

Go Placidly
Amid the Noise and Haste
And remember what peace there may be in silence.
As far as possible without surrender be on good terms with all persons.
Speak your truth quietly and
clearly; and listen to others.
Even the dull and ignorant; they
too have their story.
Avoid loud and aggressive persons, they are vexations to the spirit.
If you compare yourself with others, you may become vain and bitter;
For always there will be greater and lesser persons than yourself.
Enjoy your achievements as well as your plans.
Keep interested in your own career, however humble;
It is a real possession in the changing fortunes of time.
Exercise caution in your business affairs;
For the world is full of trickery.
But let this not blind you to what virtue there is;
Many persons strive for high ideals;
And everywhere life is full of heroism.
Be yourself. Especially, do not feign affection.
Neither be cynical about love; for in the face of all aridity and
disenchantment, it is perennial as the grass.
Take kindly the counsel of the years,
gracefully surrendering the things of youth.
Nurture strength of spirit to shield you in sudden misfortune.
But do not distress yourself with imaginings.
Many fears are born of fatigue and loneliness.
Beyond a wholesome discipline, be gentle with yourself.
You are a child of the universe; no less than the trees and the stars; you
have a right to be here.
And whether or not it is clear to you,
no doubt the universe is unfolding as it should.
Therefore be at peace with God, whatever you conceive Him to be,
And whatever your labours and aspirations, in the noisy
confusion of life.
Keep peace with your soul. With all its sham,
drudgery and broken dreams,
It is still a beautiful world.
Be careful.
Strive to be happy.

Found in Old Saint Paul's Church, Baltimore, 1692

SEX DURING PREGNANCY

SEX IN PREGNANCY is perfectly normal. In fact it can bring a new delight with it since contraception is out of the way. However, if you have previously lost a baby, been treated for infertility, or miscarried, the doctor may tell you to avoid sex when your period would have been due, or generally. If you have been asked to avoid intercourse, you can always indulge in caressing, stroking, etc. Do not feel shy to ask the doctor how long you have to avoid intercourse, since doctors may forget to say when you are past the time you are likely to miscarry. You may be asked to avoid intercourse if you have had an earlier premature labour.

If you are under great strain at work, or if you are worried about the financial responsibility of having a baby, or if you are angry about being pregnant, then you may not desire or enjoy lovemaking.

Some women feel inclined towards sex in pregnancy, while others do not. A woman's feeling should be respected. When making love certain considerations have to be kept in mind, like the growing abdomen or the increased sensitivity of the breasts. Different positions can be experimented with, in accordance with whatever is comfortable.

Men often fear that during intercourse they may in some way harm the baby. You cannot hurt the baby during intercourse. The baby is protected by the water bag and the water around it. The water acts as a shock absorber to protect the baby from accidental blows or jerks. The uterus is housed in the bony framework of the pelvic bones, which provide protection. In the mouth of the womb, called the cervix, is a plug of mucus which seals the womb and prevents infection from entering the womb. There is one precaution a couple can take to protect themselves from infection. Before intercourse the man can wash the penis and surrounding area with soap and water.

If a woman is overly anxious about her pregnancy, and her husband shares her anxiety, they will together make each other more tense. They may be so afraid of sexual arousal that they may not even lovingly touch and feel each other. A perpetual state of tension is not going to help matters. Stress of any kind is to be avoided in pregnancy. Both partners need to relax. Stroking and massaging the tension away is a good idea. Do it to each other in turns.

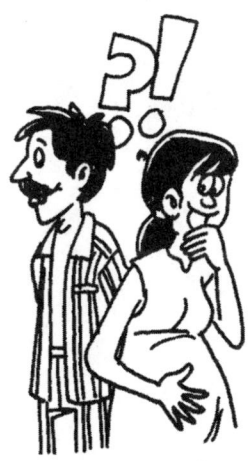

BLEEDING

Bleeding in early pregnancy may be caused if the level of your pregnancy hormone is not sufficiently high to stop your period. Such bleeding is slight, occurs for a month or a few months, when your period would have been due. It is slight with a darkish discharge, for an hour, a day or two, and there is no pain. The true significance of bleeding at the time of the period is not clear. Many women who experience it otherwise have a perfectly normal pregnancy, and a perfectly healthy baby.

However, any bleeding which occurs during pregnancy is considered a threatened abortion, and the doctor's advice must be sought. When a threatened abortion occurs, the bleeding is usually bright red or pink, which signifies that the loss is from within the uterus. When the bleeding stops, the vaginal discharge changes to dark red or brown. Normally bed rest is continued until 3 days after the brown discharge has stopped.

A threatened abortion most commonly occurs during the first three suppressed periods, that is, in the first 3 months or the 4th, 8th or 12th week of pregnancy. It could also occur in the 14th week, when the placenta takes over the production of hormones from the ovaries.

In case of threatened abortion, the doctor will advise immediate bed rest. A woman is allowed to get up only to go to the toilet. She must stay quietly in bed. She should use sanitary towels, which should be changed frequently and saved for the doctor to examine. A threatened abortion indicates an unstable pregnancy and care should be taken to rest when a period would have been due. Sexual intercourse should not take place until the doctor permits it (see p. 35).

The penis in the vagina is not threatening, as commonly believed. It is more the contractions of the uterus which are triggered off when a woman reaches orgasm that can be followed by further contractions. If you are ready to start labour or about to miscarry, these contractions may set off labour.

INTERCOURSE

It therefore follows that if your delivery is overdue this may be a more pleasant way of starting labour than a glucose drip given with a synthetic hormone added to it. Also, semen contains prostaglandin hormones which may cause the uterus to contract, or its mouth, the cervix, to soften. The greater the penetration of the penis during intercourse, the closer it will get to the cervix and bathe it with semen. It would be a good idea to place a pillow under your hips during intercourse. After your partner has ejaculated he should stay inside for a few minutes and the position must be maintained so that the prostaglandin hormone in the semen reaches the cervix. You should delay washing yourself by 10 to 15 minutes. Keep lying with the pillow under your hips.

From intercourse or from masturbation, if you have an orgasm, it causes 5 to 15 contractions, and these may be sufficient to induce labour. If you are not ready to go into labour, the effects of an orgasm in a normal stable pregnancy are not known. However, it has been suggested that when a woman reaches orgasm or a climax, and her uterus contracts, the fetus may get extra blood from the congested blood vessels.

Ordinarily, uterine contractions are quite common. They occur every few minutes throughout a woman's reproductive life from puberty to menopause, without being felt. Unless a woman is at the end of her pregnancy, unless her cervix is ready or she has a history of premature birth, uterine contractions during intercourse will not cause premature labour (see p. 89).

BREAST STIMULATION

Breast stimulation can also help start labour if your body and your baby are ready for the birth, so you need not worry about it starting labour prematurely. Stimulation of the breasts brings about contractions of the uterus, since it produces a powerful endocrine hormone by the pituitary gland, called oxytocin. A synthetic form of the same hormone in much larger doses is used by doctors to stimulate labour. If you have a tendency to start labour prematurely, avoid breast stimulation.

Breast stimulation during labour speeds up the process of labour, and in pregnancy assists in the effacement of the cervix or mouth of the womb, whereby it thins out, and softens or ripens, in preparation for birth. If a woman's delivery is overdue and labour is induced by an intra-venous drip, the labour has greater chances of ending in a normal delivery if the cervix has been softened and thinned out. Hence with breast stimulation an induced labour is more likely to end up in a normal delivery rather than in a Caesarean section. On the other hand, it may even stimulate labour to start spontaneously (see p. 88).

AFTER THE BIRTH

After the birth of the baby you will have a longish period lasting a week or several weeks. Then, if you are breastfeeding you may not have a period for several months. Even though you do not have a period, you can still conceive and become pregnant. It is therefore advisable to use a contraceptive when you resume intercourse. You can resume intercourse after 40 days or 6 weeks, since it takes that much time for the vagina to heal. You can use a lubricant like vaseline the first few times. You must consult your doctor as to which contraceptive you should use. Should intercourse take place earlier, a contraceptive like the condom can be used (see p. 165).

8   LABOUR TIME

THERE ARE 3 signs that could herald the onset of labour. These may appear by themselves or 2 may even appear together approximately 15 days before the expected date of delivery or after.

You may notice a thick mucus discharge which could be white, pink or brown in colour. Sometimes the mucus may even contain some amount of bright red blood mixed in it.

The discharge occurs from the mouth of the womb or cervix which is plugged with mucus to prevent infection from entering the womb.

A week or so before labour begins, the cervix can thin out and flatten. As this happens, the mucus plug escapes and you notice a thick lumpy mucus discharge. This discharge is a sign that your body is getting ready for the birth process. It is no cause for alarm.

The doctor would say that your cervix is now ripe, ready, or effaced.

The muscular contractions of the uterus are felt as periodic discomfort, and often referred to as pain. Initially, contractions are mild. They may feel like the mild discomfort felt at the beginning of a menstrual period. Or one may mistake them for discomfort that accompanies an upset stomach, since it is not uncommon to have diarrhoea before labour begins. On some occasions women feel it is discomfort arising from tight clothing around the waist. However, even when you switch to more comfortable clothing or lighter food, the discomfort persists. It comes and goes periodically.

When you realise this, begin to make a note of the time whenever the discomfort occurs. If you find it occurring half-hourly, you know it is real labour. It could also occur more frequently, for example, every 15 minutes. So, when it occurs at fixed intervals, you know it is real labour.

Sometimes, before labour begins you feel practice contractions or false contractions. These are contractions of the uterus in preparation for birth. Practice contractions feel similar to real contractions, but they occur at irregular intervals.

So while practice contractions have a haphazard interval between them, real contractions will have fixed, rhythmical intervals.

It is possible that after starting at periodic intervals, contractions might stop for a day or so, only to restart later. There is no harm if contractions stop. There is, at times, a slowly unfolding labour that starts and stops on and off, until it gets properly established. So you can safely stay at home until your contractions become 10 minutes apart. Once they are timed every

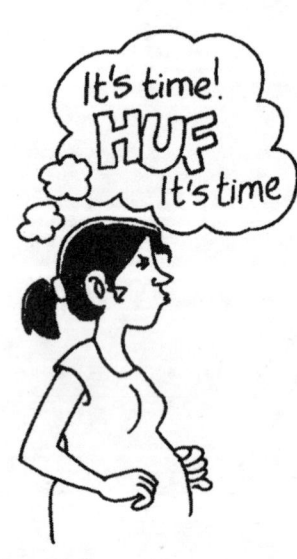

10 minutes, they are properly established and less likely to stop.

Do not panic if contractions start at 5 minute intervals.

Contractions may stop for a while when you check in to the strange atmosphere of the hospital or nursing home. If that happens, just walk around and get familiar with the place. See where the toilet is, where the nursing station is, the position of your room on the floor where you are. Stroll in the corridor and your contractions will start again as you get familiar with your environment. You could also go and have a look at the nursing home or hospital earlier, while pregnant.

After 10-minute intervals the contractions will shift to 5 minute intervals and for a short while before birth, to every 2 minutes. During birth again the interval will become 5 minutes.

FLUID LEAK

The baby is encased in the amniotic sac. Sometimes the amniotic sac bursts and all the amniotic water gushes out. About 800 ml to a litre of water may escape at once. The amniotic sac may burst before labour begins. It could happen at any time in the 9th month. Somehow, it mostly happens at night. So you could spread a rubber sheet (*momjama*) or a Quick Dry sheet across the middle of your bed.

When this happens, the amniotic fluid also sweeps out the mucus plug on its way out. The protection of the plug and the amniotic fluid is now absent. For this reason, the woman is now more susceptible to infection each time an internal examination is given. So, once the water bag bursts, doctors like to deliver the baby within 24 hours.

The common practice is to put a woman whose water bag has burst on a drip of glucose to which a synthetic hormone called syntocinon has been added in order to trigger off contractions artificially.

However, if you wait 4 to 5 hours before fixing a drip, it is possible that contractions may start spontaneously, on their own and thus eliminate the need for a drip. It would be better if this happened, since spontaneous contractions are gentler than contractions that are artificially induced.

So, if the water bag bursts, you check into a hospital, but request for the drip to be delayed by 4 to 5 hours. It is a simple request. Keeping in mind that hospital protocol says that the baby should arrive within 24 hours, waiting 4 to 5 hours still leaves an ample period of 19 to 20 hours for the birth.

On some occasions the amniotic sac may not burst, but might just trickle instead. The trickle will be clear and uncontrollable. Wear a sanitary pad and take rest at home. After some time the amniotic sac might seal itself and the trickle might stop. It might recur after some time, or it might be followed by contractions.

Go to the hospital when the contractions are 10 minutes apart, or if the trickle gets out of control and cannot be contained by a sanitary pad. The sanitary pad should be changed often to avoid infection.

WHEN URGENT MEDICAL ATTENTION IS NEEDED

A Coloured Trickle

The trickle that appears from the amniotic sac is usually clear. But if the trickle appears muddy or greenish and has a foul smell, you must get in touch with your doctor immediately. The colour in the amniotic fluid comes if the baby passes stool inside the womb, which it normally does after birth. So, once you have what is called meconium staining of the amniotic fluid you need to be under medical observation. If, along with meconium staining, there is an adverse effect on the baby's heart rate (the normal heart rate is 120 to 160 beats per minute), it would indicate a need for a Caesarean section. If the fetal heart rate is not affected, labour can progress normally, culminating in a normal delivery.

Bright Red Bleeding

If you experience bright, fresh, red bleeding like when you cut your finger, or as at the height of a period, you should be in touch with your doctor immediately. Bright, fresh, red bleeding occurs if there is placenta previa, a condition in which the placenta lies between the baby's head and the mouth of the uterus, blocking the baby's exit. Or, it could occur if the placenta detaches or peels away from the wall of the uterus. If a small portion has peeled away, it may be quite harmless, but nevertheless you will have to be under observation, to make sure it does not adversely affect the heartbeat of the baby. The normal heartbeat of the baby in labour would fluctuate between 120 and 160 beats per minute. Below 120, or above 160 are both considered fetal distress. Occasionally, a few drops of blood may escape a couple of days after intercourse, a vaginal examination by the doctor or physical exertion, like walking more than one is used to. This is quite harmless.

PRECAUTION

There is just one instance when it is better for you to lie down than be upright.

At about 36 weeks, the head of the baby fixes in the brim of the pelvic basin. In some instances, the head does not lower and fix in the pelvic basin, but remains floating above the pelvic inlet. This is called a floating head. Fairly often, a floating head fixes in the pelvic basin after labour begins.

In the last month of pregnancy when you go for weekly check-ups to your doctor, ask if the baby's head has fixed or engaged. If you have a floating head and the water bag bursts, it is possible that as all the water drains out, the umbilical cord may also be swept downwards with the water and come to lie between the baby's head and brim of the bony pelvic basin. In this case, if you remain upright, you may cause the cord to be squashed between the baby's head and the pelvis, a most undesirable situation, medically called cord prolapse. It is through the cord that the baby receives oxygen and nourishment.

When there is the rare combination of floating of the baby's head and the bursting of the water bag, you must remain lying down or adopt the knee-chest position, or go into the all-fours position.

POSITIONS TO ADOPT IN LABOUR

Once labour begins, it is best to be upright rather than lying down flat on your back. Upright would mean walking/kneeling/standing and other positions we shall discuss shortly. Being upright in labour gives the following advantages:

- The force of gravity helps in the descent of the baby. (The force of gravity is constantly pulling down things.)
- The baby with its own weight will descend through the birth canal sooner when the mother is upright, rather than when she is lying down.
- When the mother lies flat on her back, blood vessels get compressed by the weight of the uterus and the baby on the one hand and the backbone on the other. This hampers the blood flow to and from the heart, and increases the chance of distress in the mother and the baby.
- Being upright lifts the compression on the blood vessel, so that the blood flow to the mother and the baby is more efficient and both are therefore more alert and awake during birth.
- When the mother is lying down, the vagina is at an upward slant, so the baby has an uphill task before it. When the mother is upright, e.g. standing, it becomes a downward descent for the baby.
- During birth the head of the baby passes first through the top brim of the pelvic basin and then the bottom outlet of the pelvic basin. Forming part of the pelvis is the sacrum and the tail bone. These can move away as the baby comes through the outlet of the pelvis, and the space for the baby's exit increases by as much as 30%. This becomes possible only if the mother is not lying flat on her back or sitting at a 45-degree angle since these positions would press on these bones and not allow them to move.
- In 1977, a study in Birmingham Maternity Hospital compared a group of women who walked about during labour, with a group that lay down horizontally through most of labour. The results showed that in women who walked about during labour,

(i) the duration of labour was shorter;
(ii) there was less need for painkillers;
(iii) the incidence of fetal heart abnormalities was markedly lower; and
(iv) they experienced less pain.

- Further studies have revealed that:

(i) the strength or intensity of contractions is greater when women are moving about in labour; and
(ii) there is greater regularity and frequency of contractions.

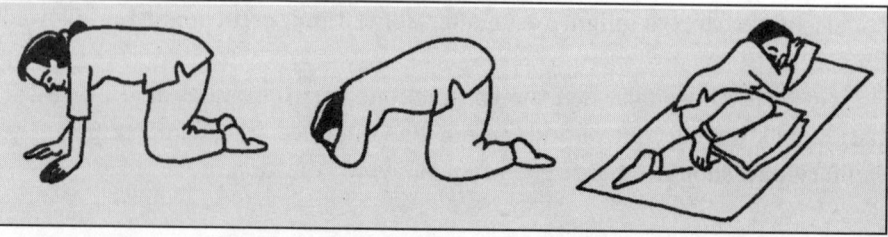

UPRIGHT POSITION FOR LABOUR

WALKING

Walking is the best position for labour. You can walk about your room, at a relaxed leisurely pace. Avoid brisk walking; it will tire you out. Stroll about, and when your contraction is felt:

- Stop walking. Stand where you are, with your feet nicely apart, balance your weight equally on both your feet. Now lean forward with your upper body totally relaxed. If you are near a piece of furniture, you can place your hands on it for support, as you lean forward. You could make a circular rotating movement with your hips, during the duration of your contraction. When the contraction is over, you can resume walking.

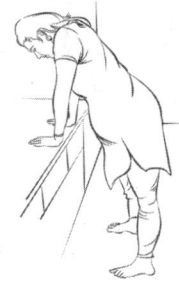

- If you happen to be near a wall when a contraction is felt, stop walking. Stand facing the wall. Place your feet apart, about one foot away from the wall. Place your palms on the wall, and lean slightly forward. Then, you may circle your hips.
- Alternatively, while you stand facing the wall, with your feet a little away from the wall, bend your arms at the elbows and place your palms on the wall, with your open palms resting on the wall. Use the back of your palms to rest your forehead on. This position helps to make the contraction stronger, especially beneficial if contractions are weak.

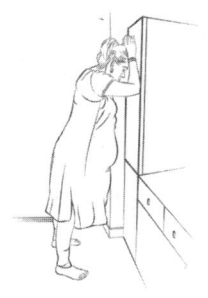

When the contraction passes, resume walking.

IN CASE THE WATER BAG BURSTS

In case the water bag bursts, and all the water gushes out altogether, the uterus is emptied of one litre of fluid. However, the water bag carries on making water which collects in the uterus and is expelled during a contraction. This would cause water running down your legs in case you are standing, or water wetting your bed in case you are sitting on a bed. To avoid wetness, you could sit on a chair with a commode, in front of the bed and lean forward on the bed when your contraction comes. This would keep you dry as the water would be collected in the commode.

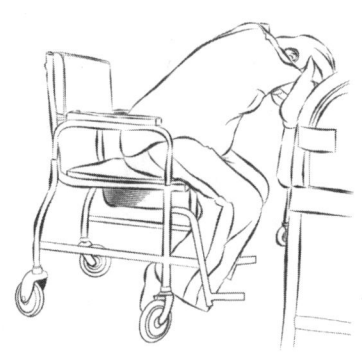

USING A DINING CHAIR

If you have labour at night when you are a bit sleepy, or if you are tired and do not want to walk or stand, this position can be used.

A dining chair is used, since it narrows on the back and has no arms. Sit facing the back of the chair, with legs on either side. Use the back to rest your head.

As you lean forward to rest your head on the back of the chair, your tail bone lifts off and moves away from the pelvic outlet, making room for the baby.

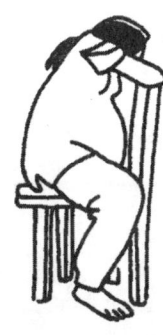

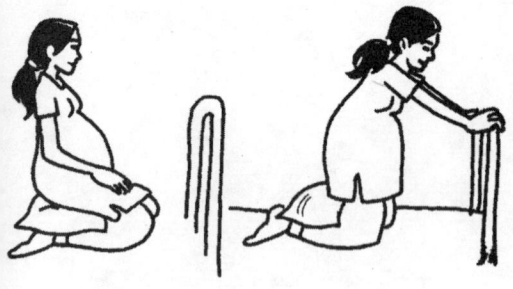

KNEELING

When you are tired of walking, another helpful position you can switch to is kneeling. You could kneel on the hospital bed.

Place a soft thick pillow on the back of your legs, that is, on the calves. Sit on the thick pillow when you are not having a contraction. When a contraction is felt, rise up on your knees, hold the headboard or footboard and bend forward or make rotating circles with your hips.

Resume sitting when the contraction passes.

BACKACHE IN LABOUR

If you feel most of the discomfort of your contraction on your lower back, you are experiencing back labour. Back labour would mean that the baby is posterior, that is, instead of facing the mother's backbone, it is facing the mother's abdomen. The back of the baby's head puts pressure on the mother's backbone, causing a low backache. Counterpressure on the lower back will relieve the discomfort.

STANDING WITH BACK TO WALL

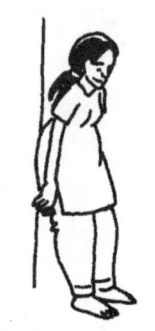

You will feel comfortable if you stand with your back to the wall and press the part of the back that hurts against the wall. To get maximum pressure on the lower back, you can hunch your shoulders forward.

ALL-FOURS POSITION

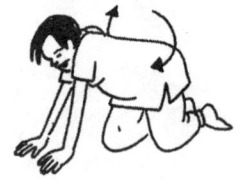

In case of a backache and a posterior baby, going on all fours and rotating the hips helps relieve the backache and rotates the baby to an anterior position. When the baby turns into an anterior position, the backache disappears.

First kneel with your knees one foot apart. Place your hands in front of you and go into the all-fours position. Rotate the hips in circles.

WHEN ON THE DRIP

The drip implies that glucose drips from a bottle through a tube, straight into your vein, through a needle that is inserted in your arm. The bottle of glucose is attached sometimes to a rod at the side of the bed; and sometimes to a rod attached to a mobile stand that has wheels. *(see p. 73).*

SITTING ON THE BED

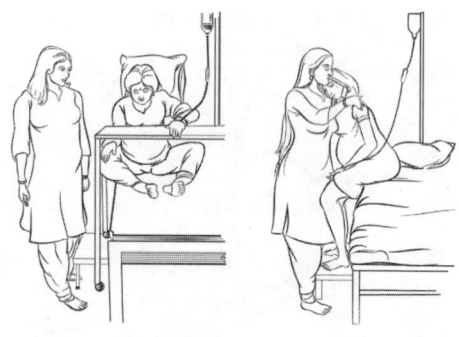

If the drip is fixed to the side of your bed, sit at the edge of the bed with your feet on the footstool. When your contraction comes, lean forward by putting a pillow on your lap and resting your elbows on them. Alternatively, lean forward and rest your head on your partner who can be standing in front of you.

You can also get off the bed and sit on a chair in front of the bed or stand in front of the bed. When the contraction comes, you can stand; hold the edge of the bed for support with your free hand.

As you stand like this, if you like, you can also move your hips in a circular motion.

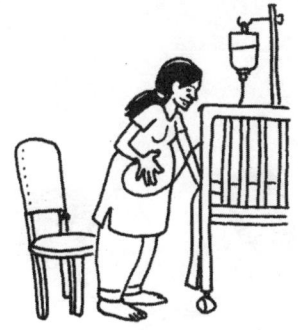

COMFORTERS

PALMING

Placing the palms on the lower abdomen and lower back of a woman who is having a contraction is of immense comfort to the labouring woman.

Just behind the muscles of the lower abdomen, the uterus contracts during a contraction. On the lower back, the joints of the pelvic structure spread apart at birth.

Hence, placing of palms on these two areas soothes the mother. It could be practised along with any position of labour.

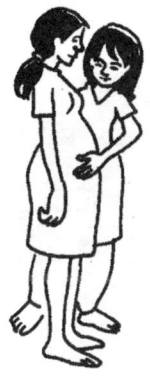

HAND SQUEEZE

Often a woman in labour desires to hold on to something or someone very tightly. If you have this urge, your partner should hold your palm with a firm, tight pressure. You should avoid gripping your partner's hand, so that you do not waste energy and strength while doing so; and you do not tense your body. Remove rings before trying this, they could hurt.

Your partner's thumb should be placed at the back of your hand. The remaining 4 fingers should fold on the back of the hand from the opposite side. The grip should be firm. You should tell your partner if you want to increase the pressure or have it lessened.

EFFLEURAGE

The skin and muscles of the abdomen are very tense during a uterine contraction. A light massage or brushing will lessen this tension.

Effleurage is a light moving of your fingertips on your lower abdomen, that is, between the navel and the pubic hair. Place the fingertips of both hands on either side of the navel. Make circles by moving fingers lightly in a circular motion from the centre of the abdomen, outwards, towards the hips. Then down towards the pubic hairline and up towards the navel.

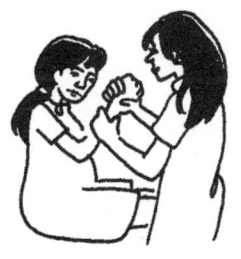

If you are on the drip and one hand is immobilized, you can massage with the fingertips of one hand, from side to side; that is, from one hip to the other, across the lower abdomen. Your partner could do this massage for you.

The fingertips should move in light strokes, rubbing should be avoided. The lighter the strokes, the better. It should be done simultaneously with breathing exercise. Apply talcum powder as needed.

It is more soothing if the stroking is done with one's flat fingernails, so one can fold one's fingertips towards the palm and use the surface of one's nails to do the stroking.

This kind of stroking can also be done on the mother's back in a 'V' shape.

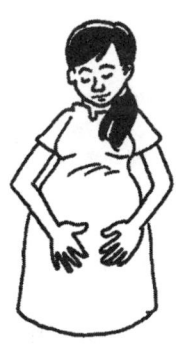

Stroking also enhances the release of the hormone oxytocin which is of immense benefit to mother and baby.

LEG MASSAGE

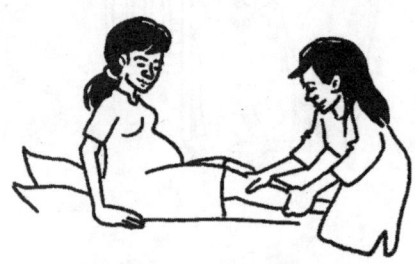

If you feel your legs are weak or shaky, a massage moving firmly upwards from above the ankles, on the sides of your legs, will feel good. You can use talcum powder so that your fingers run smoothly and are not hampered by perspiration.

If you feel shaky on the thighs, this massage can be done from above the knees, on the inner and outer sides of the thighs. Sometimes this massage could be done after the birth of the baby.

FOR A BACKACHE

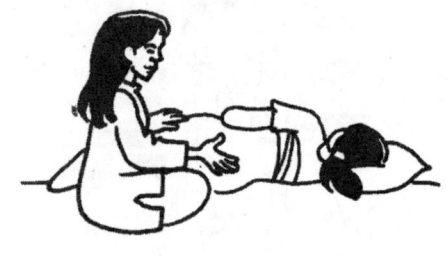

In labour, a slight discomfort in the back is common. Backache is more pronounced in the case of back labour or a posterior baby, when the discomfort of labour is concentrated more in the lower back than in the lower abdomen.

BACK MASSAGE

Lie on your side. Take a pillow under your head and another pillow between your knees.

Your partner should sit facing your back. With one hand he can hold your hip, so that you do not have to brace yourself, and with the other hand, locate the flat, hard surface of your lower back, just above your hips. Once located, the palm should be pressed on the spot. Then rotate the palm clockwise and anti-clockwise. This massage can be practised during pregnancy too, in case of a backache.

Since a great amount of pressure is applied by the palm, it helps if the person massaging supports the elbow of the massaging hand on the thigh, or any other part of the body, for instance, on the stomach. This will reduce the strain on the shoulder, and make it possible to do it for a longer period of time.

However, if tiredness sets in, your partner can instead sit back-to-back with you.

During a contraction stand and have your partner place one hand on your lower abdomen, just above the pubic hairline, while the other hand should be placed on the lower back, above the hips. No pressure is required to be exerted with the hands. The hands are to be placed gently on these two places. After a contraction, with both hands in place, exhale, then let go of your abdomen. Relax your abdomen towards the hand. Relax your pelvic floor. Leave the pelvic floor relaxed as though you are passing urine. Imagine your pelvis is opening up, and having passed through it your baby is now coming through your relaxed vagina. Relax your hips and buttocks. Relax your inner thigh and your outer thigh.

BACK TO BACK

You should continue lying on your side, as for the back massage above. Your partner should sit against your lower back, with a straight back, exactly where the flatness of your back is. That is, leaning on you should be avoided, or else you will feel that you might tumble over.

At times, if your partner is male, just this sitting is adequate. However, if you feel the pressure is less, your partner should lean forward, cross both palms at the back, place them on your lower back and straighten again. This will add to the pressure and bring greater comfort.

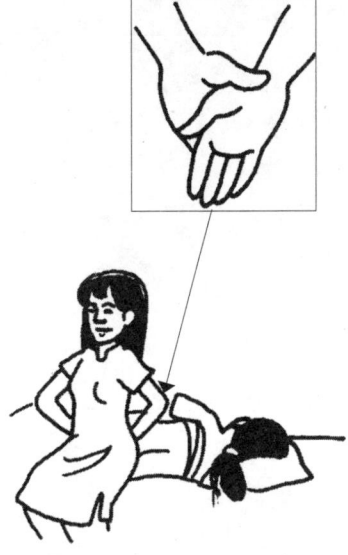

9

BREATHING AND RELAXATION FOR LABOUR

IGNORANCE-FEAR-TENSION-PAIN SYNDROME

THE UTERUS IS made up of strong muscles whose action causes it to open and let the baby pass first through its opening (cervix), and then through the vaginal passage into the doctor's hands. Childbirth therefore depends largely on the efficient working of the muscles of the uterus and the vagina.

Muscles in our body are of 2 types, voluntary muscles and the involuntary muscles. Voluntary muscles are those over which we have direct control, the muscles of the arms and legs, for instance. Involuntary muscles are those over which we have no direct control, like the muscles of our heart or uterus.

If a woman is tense during labour, her uterine muscles will also get tense and perform with great difficulty, because tension in the body is infectious; it passes from one muscle to the other. However, if she is relaxed, her uterine muscles will work unhampered, and with each contraction they will get closer to complete dilation of the cervix, so that the woman will have a shorter, less painful labour.

This is called the ignorance-fear-tension-pain syndrome. That is, ignorance of how the body functions during childbirth causes a fear of the unknown. Fear causes tension, which in turn leads to rigid abdominal muscles, more pain and longer labour. Whereas, if you eliminate ignorance, by understanding the physiology of birth, you eliminate the fear of the unknown. Without fear, tension will be absent, leading to easy muscle action, so that your body functions as nature intended it to, without being hampered by tension.

QUICK RELAXATION IN LABOUR

Relax the lower abdomen, pelvic floor, hips and buttocks and your thighs, each time a contraction is over. Then go on to general relaxation.

There are certain points in the body where tension tends to accumulate. If you work at relaxing these points, you will quickly achieve relaxation.

- Relax your forehead. Stop frowning. Pinch your eyebrows and stroke your forehead.
- Relax your jaw. A relaxed jaw is a relaxed vagina.

- Separate your teeth and let your tongue be static in the middle of your mouth.
- Relax your shoulders.
- Relax your elbows. Loosen them and move them away from your body.
- Relax your hands.
- Relax your feet.

If you find it difficult to relax any of these points, have your partner massage them for you. For instance, your partner can massage your shoulders, face or feet, to help you relax. Practise this daily, so that you use it with ease during labour.

Each time a contraction is over, go into relaxation. During a contraction, the uterus is partially deprived of blood and oxygen. Relaxation after the contraction sends a plentiful supply of this life-giving fluid to the uterus. When the body is relaxed, the muscles in the body use a minimum of energy, and oxygen-enriched blood reaches the uterus and the baby, ensuring a healthier and alert baby. Also, using the rest periods between contractions to your maximum advantage will not allow tension to build up and accumulate in your body, keeping you relaxed right through.

When a contraction occurs, concentrate on keeping your face relaxed. If you keep your face relaxed, automatically the rest of your body will also become relaxed. Tension anywhere in the body will show on the face.

BREATHING FOR LABOUR

Properly regulated breathing during labour will help take away the pain of labour.

Breathing has to be practised regularly before delivery, so that you can slip into breathing effortlessly when you go into labour.

CONDITIONED REFLEX

Reflexes are instantaneous and involuntary responses to stimuli. There are 2 types of reflexes. The inborn reflex, e.g. blinking to protect the eyes from a blow, or the conditioned reflex of feeling hunger at meal-time.

As an inborn reflex, a dog will salivate if meat is put in his mouth. If, however, the introduction of meat is preceded by the ringing of a bell, and this process is repeated several times, the dog ends up salivating when just the bell is rung and no meat is given. Hence, a conditioned reflex has been established, which associates food with the sound of the bell and so determines the response of salivation.

In the same way, breathing regularly practised for labour establishes a pathway to the brain which associates breathing with labour. When labour actually sets in, the brain determines the response of breathing.

BREATHING FOCUS

Breathing during labour brings about a focus of activity in one part of the brain, from where it has a tendency to develop and spread. For instance, a pupil paying attention to what the teacher is saying is not aware of noise in the street, because the attention he is paying to the teacher's lecture localises the focus of activity in his brain, and becomes surrounded by a zone of inhibition into which all the stimuli from surrounding noises drain. In the same way, a toothache, which is hardly noticed when one is busy with some important activity, becomes stabbing during inactivity.

The aim of preparation for labour by learning breathing patterns is to reinforce to its maximum the inhibition of the brain, by bringing about a focus on breathing activity during labour.

The strength of inhibition brought about by your focus on breathing activity will depend on the strength of your focus on your breathing patterns. This in turn will depend on the work and practice you have put into the development of this focus. The success of your labour is therefore in your hands.

This is stressed by the French doctor, Lamaze, in the psychoprophylactic method of childbirth, based on Pavlov's experiments carried out in Russia.

According to Dr Lamaze, in the book *Painless Childbirth* (New York, 1972), 'a woman learns how to give birth the same way she learns how to swim or write or read—and she does so without pain.'

BREATHING PATTERNS

DEEP CLEANSING BREATH

Before any kind of breathing is practised, first take a deep cleansing breath. That is, you fully fill and empty your lungs.

Breathe in deeply through the nose and let it out through the mouth. Take this breath at the beginning and at the end of a breathing practice.

WAIST-LEVEL BREATHING

Breathe in deeply through the nose, and breathe out slowly through your mouth, as though you were trying to flicker the flame of a burning candle held at arm's length, with the air that you are exhaling.

Practise a few times.

Now, do your quick relaxation, then practise this breathing for 30 seconds, beginning and ending with a deep cleansing breath.

The number of waist-level breaths should be between 4 and 6 in 30 seconds. If it is more than 6 you are breathing too fast. Slow down your breathing accordingly.

CHEST-LEVEL BREATHING

Place your hands at your chest, below your collarbone. In addition, you can have your partner place one hand at the bra level on your back. Now breathe in and out through your mouth up to your hands, a shallow, slow, and gentle breath. The breath in, is short upto the collarbone; whereas the breath out is slower and longer.

So that your mouth does not get dry, place the tip of your tongue on the roof of the mouth.

Practise a few times.

Do your quick relaxation. Practise this breathing for 30 seconds, beginning and ending with a deep cleansing breath.

Count the number of chest-level breaths practised, without counting the deep cleansing breaths. The number should be between 10 and 12 breaths in 30 seconds. If you exceed 12 breaths, slow down your breathing.

JAW-LEVEL BREATHING, 'OUT'

The jaw-level breathing entails simply saying the word 'Out' with a stress on the 'T'. Do not worry about your breathing, it will take care of itself as you say the word.

Practise a few times.

Do your quick relaxation. Practise the breathing for 30 seconds, beginning and ending with a deep cleansing breath.

You could get between 20 and 25 breaths in 30 seconds, not counting the deep cleansing breaths. If you exceed 25 breaths, slow down breathing.

Now you are ready to do a breathing practice. Let us imagine you are having a contraction which slowly builds up to a peak and then tapers away.

> **PRECAUTION**
>
> If you ever feel dizzy while doing the breathing practices, cover your nose and mouth with your palms and blow out once. Then breathe normally. This will re-establish the proper balance of oxygen and carbon dioxide in your body and relieve dizziness if it is experienced.

BREATHING PRACTICE		
Your partner says	You do	Duration
Contraction begins	One deep cleansing breath and waist-level breathing.	15 Secs
It is getting stronger	Chest-level breathing	15 Secs
Still stronger	Out breathing	15 Secs
It's going away	Chest-level breathing	15 Secs
Further away	Waist-level breathing	15 Secs
It's gone	One deep cleansing breath	

Practise this a few times with verbal instructions.

Thereafter we will simulate a contraction, that is, create a mock contraction. To do so, we will practise with pressure on the wrist.

At the inner wrists the nerves are sensitive. By exerting pressure on them, according to the breathing, we acquaint the nerves with the message that the greater the pressure, the shallow the breathing. Conversely, the less the pressure, or the discomfort, the deeper the breathing. For instance, when you walk, you do not breathe as shallow as you do when you are running.

In labour the pressure will not be given on the wrist in this manner. When labour begins, the nerve endings on the uterus will send similar messages to the brain as contractions progress. The brain will automatically respond

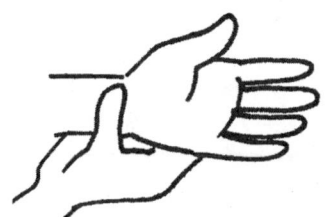

to greater discomfort with shallower breathing, due to the earlier practice with pressure on the wrist.

Your partner should hold your wrist, with four fingers underneath and the thumb on the centre of the wrist on the top. Then, your partner should exert pressure on the wrist in accordance with the verbal instructions, during a breathing practice.

Your partner says	And...
Contraction begins	rests the thumb lightly on the wrist
It's getting stronger	exerts a little pressure on the wrist
Still stronger	exerts maximum pressure
It's going away	reduces the pressure slightly
Further away	returns to resting the thumb lightly on the wrist, firm grip on the wrist
It's gone	releases pressure totally

Do 5 rounds of breathing practice daily. Remember to do your quick relaxation before you begin, and repeat the relaxation after each breathing practice. You can practise on waking in the morning or before sleeping at night.

In labour you will do whatever breathing you feel like doing. What you eventually use will depend on whether you are naturally a deep or shallow breather; whether your labour is artificially induced or a natural labour, whether you are sleepy or awake, etc.

CONCENTRATION BREATHING

Close your eyes and concentrate on the space between your eyebrows. Imagine you see there the image of someone you love/worship, or an image of something beautiful, like a beautiful sunset you might have seen recently, or a favourite picture.

Concentrate on the image and leave your mouth open slightly. Breathe naturally and effortlessly through your mouth.

CONCENTRATION BREATHING CAN BE USED AS DISTRACTION BREATHING

If you are being given an internal examination, take a deep cleansing breath and go into concentration breathing, leaving your pelvic floor muscle relaxed as when passing urine.

If you are distracted by another patient, a member of the staff, or by well-meaning relatives, go into your concentration breathing. It will remove you from your immediate environment and you will not feel disturbed. You can couple your concentration breathing with the other breathing levels, that is, as you do waist-level, chest-level and 'Out' breathing, you can close your eyes and concentrate on your image at the same time.

If you are wheeled into the operation theatre and want to take your attention off the frightening equipment around you, concentration breathing will help.

When an injection is being given, or when the drip is being fixed on your arm, do the concentration breathing.

NOT-PUSHING BREATHING

The old wives' tale which says that one must push the moment labour begins, is false. Physically pushing out the baby should be done only at birth. Before birth, both lips of the cervix have to move away from the baby's head.

Just before the birth of the baby, while one lip could have moved away, the other could still be covering part of the baby's head. If you push prematurely, it could cause the baby's head to hit against the unopened lip of the cervix, causing swelling and tenderness, or pain.

You might experience a desire to bear down and push the baby out, in the middle of a contraction. It is important to immediately inform the staff how you feel, and not bear down until the staff or the doctor says that you can do so. To avoid bearing down do the following breathing:

2 shallow pants	Blow
The shallow pants are like chest-level breathing, done quickly.	
2 shallow pants	Blow
2 shallow pants	Blow

If the urge to push is very strong, you may need to blow out several times in a row. That is:

2 shallow pants	Blow. Blow. Blow.

Occasionally, some women who have had induced labour have used this breathing during labour.

TRANSITION BREATHING

Transition is an intense period before the birth of the baby. The cervix dilates to a total of 10 cm to permit the passing of the baby's head. During transition the cervix could be about 8 cm dilated (10 cm is full dilation). That is, the dilation of the cervix is soon going to be complete and the expulsion of the baby through the vagina is going to begin.

There is soon going to be a transition from the first stage of labour to the second stage. Transition can last from two to three hours approximately. It is a sign that birth will happen soon.

You might just sail through the transition without feeling a thing. On the other hand, you might feel cold or hot or nauseous during this phase.

During transition your contractions are closest together. They could come

2 minutes apart and can be sharp long ones, lasting a whole minute. The 'Out' and concentration breathing could be most suitable at this stage.

Typical of this stage is a premature desire to push the baby out. If you push before the cervix is fully dilated, the cervix can become swollen and resist opening up.

Transition is characterised by a release of the stress hormones that are released to help the mother push the baby out. Therefore a negative change of mood could happen. You might suddenly feel angry or discouraged or helpless or in need of a painkiller. You might be angry with the hospital set-up or your partner. You might feel discouraged, that you've been in labour for so many hours, 'nothing is happening!' You might feel helpless at your situation and your inability to run away from it.

This is also the time when you might be offered a painkiller. Medication at this stage is best avoided, as it can slow down the birth process and require the use of instruments at birth, that is, the use of forceps, or the use of vacuum extraction.

It's important to remember at this point that this must be transition and therefore a sign that you are very close to birth.

Some women find the hand squeeze comforting at this stage, whereas others do not like being touched. This is the time when a woman internalises and knows she has to make a go of it all by herself. She aligns with the process her body is undergoing. It helps to know that this is a short and intense phase.

Dr Odent feels that at this moment the spouse assisting the woman in labour can exit the room. He feels the presence of the husband at birth can negatively affect the romance in the relationship post the birth of the baby.

PUSHING BREATHING

When dilation of the cervix is complete to 10 cm or 5 fingers, and the baby is being pushed out through the birth canal or vagina, the second stage of labour has begun. At this time contractions slow down to being 5 minutes part.

At this stage, you will be taken to the delivery room. The delivery room has a special table on which you will be made to lie, with your legs apart. Your legs may be supported by stirrups. Alternatively, you will be told to place your legs bent at the knees and your feet placed flat on the table. Some fancy hospitals have special delivery beds, on which mothers are in an upright kind of position at birth, sitting at a 45-degree angle.

They may have these beds in LDRs (Labour, Delivery and Recovery Rooms). In an LDR the mother is not shifted to the delivery room. The bed she is on is adjustable. It is adjusted for birth by dismantling half the bed and raising the head end. The lower part of the bed on the foot side has foot rests for the mother's feet.

On the side there may be handlebars for the mother to hold, as she sits at a 45-degree angle and births the baby.

Whatever bed you may be on, when the doctor tells you to push, you can do the breathing described below.

During practice, either lie down using 2 pillows under your head, or sit with your back supported by the wall and your legs bent at the knees and feet flat on the floor, then take:

1 waist-level breath (inhale through the nose up to your waist and blow out through pursed lips).

Take a 2nd waist-level breath, and hold the back of your thighs.

Take a 3rd waist-level breath, and after inhaling, hold your breath, and incline your chin towards your chest.

While you hold your breath, with chin to chest, whatever pressure you apply at the time of birth is not concentrated in the neck, and is automatically diverted towards the pelvic floor.

When you cannot hold your breath any longer, it is a sign that your body needs more oxygen, so exhale and quickly inhale and resume holding your breath.

Do not physically apply pressure downwards as when you are constipated. Physical application of pressure is to be practised only at the time of actual birth. When practising, just practise holding your breath, and while holding your breath, release your pelvic floor as when passing urine.

So when you feel the start of a contraction and are told to push, you do:

1st waist-level, and do nothing else.

2nd waist-level, and hold the back of your thighs.

3rd waist-level. Hold the breath. Simultaneously incline chin towards chest, and relax the pelvic floor.

Then, if the contraction is not yet over, exhale, and immediately inhale and hold the breath. Keep holding your breath till the contraction lasts.

When the contraction is over, raise your chin back up, relax by making your muscles limp, and switch to concentration breathing.

If you are doing this in a lying down position, you will need to raise your head, neck and shoulders as you grab the back of your thighs, when you take the second waist-level breath.

After you deliver the baby, it's best to have the baby wiped and placed on your chest. This can be done after a caesarean section also. When the baby is placed on the mother's chest the stress hormone release stops, and the mother and baby both start to release oxytocin, the hormone that promotes mutual bonding and facilitates a successful start to breastfeeding. Further, it promotes a feeling of security in the baby, since the mother's breasts smell of the amniotic fluid that the baby had existed in, inside the uterus. This feeling of security and love stays with the baby throughout its life. It's a 'life insurance' that cannot be bought later!

10 INDUCED LABOUR

THE ESTIMATED DATE OF DELIVERY

THE ESTIMATED DATE of delivery is not a date of appointment. It is simply a date arrived at by a rough calculation, to estimate the average duration of pregnancy. A pregnancy might exceed it or terminate before it. Studies show that only 4 to 5% of babies arrive on the estimated date of delivery.

On an average a pregnancy lasts 280 days, 40 weeks, or 9 months and 7 days, after the first day of the last menstrual period. There is no disadvantage to the baby if the birth takes place anytime spontaneously between 38 and 42 weeks of pregnancy.

To calculate a woman's estimated date of delivery, one takes into account the last menstrual period before her pregnancy. Suppose it began on 25 March, one would count 7 days on and arrive at 1 April. Then one would count backwards 3 months, that is 1 March, 1 February, 1 January. The estimated date of delivery would be 1 January. This is a short-cut to counting 280 days from a fixed date.

However, 40 weeks or 280 days is merely an average. The maturity of the baby could occur anywhere from the 38th week to the 42nd week.

The actual birth date of the baby will be influenced by the menstrual cycle of the mother. Some women have a 25 or a 28-day menstrual cycle, while others may have a 35 or 40 day menstrual cycle. Ovulation and conception generally occur about 14 days before the onset of the next period. A woman with a 25-day cycle will have conceived sooner and will deliver sooner than a woman with a 35-day cycle, since the gap between her periods is shorter than the gap of a woman who has a 35-day cycle. A lengthy cycle would mean birth beyond the due date. In calculating the estimated date of delivery it is important for a woman to be sure of her dates.

A woman with a regular cycle will deliver more predictably than one with an irregular cycle. A twin pregnancy could be shorter by 3 weeks. Triplet and quadruplet pregnancies could be shorter still. However, it is better to retain the pregnancy until full term, so it is important to avoid physical stress in the last few weeks of a multiple pregnancy. It is better for the babies.

A woman who has been on the pill may conceive without having regular periods. It is a good idea to use some other contraceptive after the pill has been stopped and have at least 3 regular periods before conception.

Although the exact reason why labour starts when it does is not known, there is a great amount of evidence that shows that the fetus, when it is ready for existing outside the womb, produces a hormone which leads to the onset of labour.

WHEN LABOUR IS INDUCED

Induction is a way of artificially stimulating the uterus into labour contractions, with the intention of controlling the birth of the baby.

Sometimes labour may be induced for the sake of your convenience or the doctor's. Your convenience could be your desire to rejoin work on a particular date, to time a transfer of residence to your convenience, or to attend a wedding or some social function. The doctor's convenience may be a plan to attend a long-awaited medical conference or a long-planned vacation. Or it could be the timing of the birth at a time when most medical staff are on duty.

For an induction to be successful, the baby must be full-term and term size, with its head pressing down at the mouth of the womb, which should be soft, short and partially dilated. If these conditions are absent, the induction can terminate in a Caesarean section.

As you go past your due date you might begin to get anxious about when the birth will take place. Your anxiety can be made worse by people who phone and ask what news there is. The doctor may have told you that if you go past your due date labour may be induced.

Doctors are divided in their opinion as to when labour should be induced for post-maturity. When everything is normal, some doctors would not mind allowing a pregnancy up to 42 weeks. Each pregnancy should be treated as an individual case. Certain factors like hypertension or toxaemia would warrant an induction.

PLANNED CAESAREAN

If one is planning to have a Caesarean section because the position of the baby is breech, or because you are having twins, it is better to wait for labour to begin spontaneously, and then have the Caesarean. That is the time the baby is ready to live independently, to breathe independently, suck and regulate its body temperature.

Such a baby is less likely to be traumatized from being delivered too early, and is more likely to have optimal brain development.

According to Dr Lackritz, chief of maternal and infant health at the National Centers for Disease Control and Prevention, Atlanta, USA, 'The baby's brain at 35 weeks gestation weighs only two-thirds of what it will weigh at 39 to 40 weeks.' She further adds, 'During the last few weeks of pregnancy, vital organs like the brain, lungs and liver are still developing. There are also fewer vision and hearing problems among babies born at full term. If there is no medical complication, the healthiest outcome for both mother and infant is delivery at 40 weeks.'

DIFFERENT METHODS OF INDUCTION

CASTOR OIL

Earlier, at full term women used to be given castor oil, and the next day labour would be triggered off if they were really ready to go into labour. Sometimes it was coupled with a hot bath and enema.

About 25 to 50 ml of castor oil can be whisked into a hot sweetened cup of milk and drunk by the woman a night before she is scheduled for induction of labour.

If her body is ready to go into labour she could start labour spontaneously the next day. If her body is not ready for labour the castor oil would act as a laxative. She would have a loose stool and settle down.

SWEEPING AND STRETCHING OR STRIPPING

Just before or during labour, when the cervix is lax, this procedure can be carried out.

While an internal vaginal examination is being given, the membranes of the water bag are swept off the wall of the uterus around its mouth, by the fingers, and the cervix is stretched by the fingers.

This speeds up labour. It may be followed by induction.

GEL OR PESSARY

A gel or pessary containing prostaglandin hormone could be placed at the mouth of the womb or cervix during a vaginal examination. As it melts and comes in contact with the cervix, it causes it to soften in preparation for birth.

ARTIFICIAL RUPTURE OF MEMBRANES

Artificial rupture of membranes, often referred to as ARM, consists of artificially rupturing the membrane of the bag of water surrounding the baby in the womb. It is done during an internal vaginal examination.

If the membranes are not made to rupture, they might rupture spontaneously during the course of labour, more typically when dilation of the cervix has been completed. In some instances the membranes may rupture at birth.

After the bag is made to burst during labour, the contractions will increase in intensity. ARM speeds up labour, and is one way of inducing contractions. It is useful in prolonged labour with little progress.

It may be resorted to when the fetal heart shows signs of distress. The breaking of the water then facilitates the doctor to check the water for meconium staining. If the water is coloured green or muddy from the baby's stool, it is a sign of distress, for the baby normally should pass the first stool after birth, not in the uterus.

Dr Ian Donald says in his *Practical Obstetric Problems:* 'With very few exceptions, intact membranes mean an intact mother and an intact baby.'

There are also fewer chances of cord prolapse when the membranes are intact. Cord prolapse occurs when the cord, on being swept down with the water, comes to lie between the bones of the pelvis and the baby's head, causing distress to the baby. Pressure on the cord is another possibility when the rupture of membranes causes powerful contractions that exert pressure on the cord and reduce the flow of blood and oxygen to the baby.

When the membranes are intact there are fewer chances of infection.

Also, intact membranes mean that even hydrostatic pressure is applied to the whole fetal surface, so that the birth experience is gentler for the baby.

When a baby is born with membranes intact, there is less likelihood of the uterus closing up after the birth of the baby, and before the delivery of the placenta.

Keeping all these points in mind, routine ARM is most undesirable.

ARM is also sometimes referred to as ROM or Rupture of Membranes. Sometimes it can happen prematurely and spontaneously before the mother completes her full term of pregnancy. At such times it may be referred to as PROM i.e. Premature Rupture of Membranes.

If the membranes are ruptured artificially while giving an internal examination it is referred to as AROM or Artificial Rupture of Membranes.

When the membranes rupture spontaneously at full term it is referred to as SROM or Spontaneous Rupture of Membranes. People often refer to the rupture of membranes as 'my water bag burst' or 'the water bag broke'.

INTRAMUSCULAR INJECTION

An injection of pitocin may be given in the arm or in the hip. Pitocin speeds up labour when contractions become lax.

Once labour is established a course of 3 to 5 epidocin injections may be given to speed up the opening up or dilation of the cervix.

INTRAVENOUS DRIP

The commonly used procedure for induction these days is to trigger off labour with the use of a synthetic form of the oxytocin hormone, which in natural labour is secreted by the mother's pituitary gland and makes the uterus contract. The artificial form of oxytocin, called syntocin, is added to a bottle of glucose solution and introduced straight into the mother's bloodstream through a drip attached to her arm. A fine needle is inserted into a vein in the arm and kept in place.

Doctors like to use the drip because the glucose gives you energy without your needing to eat anything. So if a Caesarean section is needed, your stomach is likely to be empty as needed for the administration of general anesthesia. If you eat, there is the risk that while under anaesthesia you might vomit and inhale the contents into your lungs.

However, if epidural/spinal anesthesia is used, the mother is awake through the process, as the lower part of her body is anesthetized with a local anesthetic. So in case of epidural/spinal anesthesia this risk of aspiration of the vomit does not occur.

The energy you can get from glucose will be useful if you have had a long-drawn labour and become tired. So while in labour you can also drink glucose dissolved in water, when you begin to feel tired.

Once a drip is set up, any drug apart from syntocin can be introduced into the bloodstream through it, without your being aware of it. If you are on the drip, each time the bottle is changed ask what it is. The bottle would have 'Synto' written on it to indicate the syntocin hormone.

Routine use of the drip is best avoided. It does not necessarily result in dilation or progress of labour. It will make you immobile in labour, confining you to the bed. It will also make labour sharper and stronger, unnecessarily adding to your discomfort.

INDICATIONS FOR INTRAVENOUS DRIP

There are times, such as prolonged labour, when a drip may be needed. Labour may be triggered off by the intravenous glucose drip in certain conditions like toxaemia, very high blood pressure, diabetes, prolonged pregnancy beyond 42 weeks. Sometimes it is used if considerable time has elapsed after the water bag has burst and labour has not begun on its own.

If you happen to need the drip, remember to pass urine frequently while on it, to avoid your bladder getting very full. Request for the glucose bottle to be fixed on a stand with wheels, rather than for it to be fixed to the side of your bed. That would allow you to go to the toilet when required and also allow general mobility. If the drip is fixed to the side of your bed, request for a long tube so that you can turn over and move about in bed. If it is short, you will feel trapped. Avoid putting weight on the arm on which the drip is fixed.

HOME INDUCTIONS

BREAST STIMULATION

If your partner sucks at your nipples, or either of you stroke and massage the nipples and the breasts, it will stimulate the release of oxytocin hormone in your body, and if your body is ready, over a period of time it can cause labour to start. Applying a warm cloth to your breasts can have the same effect. Fifteen days before your estimated date of delivery, you can take a mug of warm water and dip two face towels in it. Wring the water out of them and apply them on the front of the breast, so that they cover the nipple, and areola. This will cause you to feel a pleasant warm sensation. When you feel this, remove the towels and dip them in water again and re-apply them on the breast. Do 6 times altogether.

Repeat 4 times a day. Morning, afternoon, evening and night

At the Letter man Army Medical Center in San Francisco, 2 groups of 100 women each in the 39th week of pregnancy were instructed to rub both nipples gently between their fingertips for an hour, three times daily. By the 42nd week 89 breast stimulators had gone into spontaneous labour, as compared with *77* non-breast stimulators in the other groups. Also, only

5 breast stimulators had unripe cervixes as compared to 17 in the other group (see p. 67).

INTERCOURSE

If your delivery is overdue and the doctor says induction may be considered, it is a good idea to indulge in intercourse. Seminal fluid is rich in prostoglandin hormones which are known to ripen the cervix and stimulate contractions. The cervix is thus affected locally and labour begins more naturally as compared to being put on the intravenous drip in the hospital (see p. 67).

PROLONGED PREGNANCY

A pregnancy can go 14 days over the estimated date of delivery. However, most obstetricians do not like the pregnancy to prolong beyond 7 to 10 days after the estimated date of delivery. If pregnancy extends upto 43 weeks, doctors are concerned that:

- Beyond this time the placenta begins to get fibrous and its efficiency to nourish the baby decreases.
- The measure of amniotic fluid dwindles as the baby gets bigger, so it could result in a dry labour.
- The cranial or head bones harden and no moulding of the head takes place during birth.
- Whether labour needs to be induced or not depends on the baby's well-being. The baby's well-being can be assessed in the following ways:

FETAL HEART RATE

If the fetal heart rate is normal, it is a sign that all is well with the baby. The average fetal heart rate is between 120 to 160 beats per minute. It is healthy for it to fluctuate during a contraction. Fluctuation indicates that the baby is responding to stimuli, which is a good sign. In some countries the normal heart rate of the baby in labour is considered to be 110 to 150 beats per minute. Oftentimes the heart rate may go above or below the limits for a brief moment and correct itself in minutes.

PLACENTAL INSUFFICIENCY I.U.G.R.

Placental insufficiency will be suspected if the doctor feels that the baby is not growing, since the size of the uterus will be smaller than it should be. This could occur in underweight, malnourished women, in women prone to drug abuse, women with high blood pressure, chronic kidney disease. It could also happen in women prone to pre-eclampsia, heart, lung or gastro-intestinal disorders, and women suffering from infection.

According to the book *Obstetrics and the Newborn*, 1997, in case of I.U.G.R., the second baby is likely to fare much better than the first baby.

If the doctor suspects slow fetal growth, improve your diet. If you are already eating well, rest. Rest encourages blood flow to the uterus and the

The growth of the baby is estimated not by the largeness of the mother's abdomen but by the height of the growing uterus. It is only in about the 4th month that the pregnancy begins to show externally, as the abdomen enlarges. A few weeks before delivery the uterus may drop or lower as the baby's head goes into the pelvis.

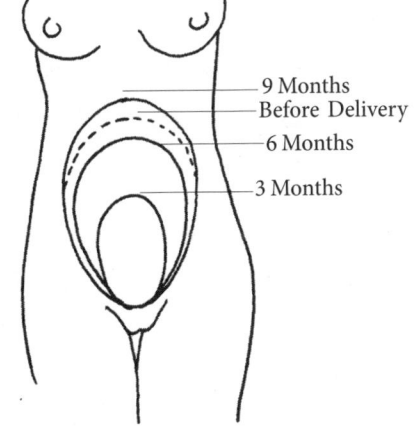

baby, and after bed rest a sudden spurt in the baby's growth may be noticed at the next check-up. As you rest, favour lying on your side to lying on your back, it will encourage greater blood and oxygen supply to the baby. Lying on the left side encourages optimum oxygen supply to the baby. Avoid a smoke-filled atmosphere.

If this does not help the baby's growth, the baby may be delivered by a Caesarean section or labour may be induced, depending on what the doctor thinks best.

DIABETIC MOTHER

Some women may develop diabetes in pregnancy, while some others may be diabetic to begin with. Diabetes that starts in pregnancy is called gestational diabetes, and is more likely to occur in the last 3 months of pregnancy. A high glucose level in early pregnancy could mean that the mother was diabetic before pregnancy without realising it. Most women who develop gestational diabetes will find that their glucose levels return to normal after delivery. However, gestational diabetes could return with the next pregnancy. The possibility can be reduced by following a healthy diet and not putting on too much weight.

Frequently, pregnant women may show glucose in their urine without having diabetes, as in pregnancy the resistance level at which glucose spills into the urine comes down. A glucose tolerance test can identify whether the woman has an unusually low renal threshold, but not diabetes, or whether she has diabetes.

Women who are diabetic before becoming pregnant have an excess of blood sugar which the baby absorbs and tends to become very large. The doctor will recommend a restriction of sweet foods to these mothers.

A diabetic mother may be induced early so that the baby does not get so big that a safe vaginal delivery is impossible. Despite its large size, the baby may not be mature and may need special care after birth. Sometimes if the cervix is not soft and ready to open up, a Caesarean section may be performed.

Whether you develop diabetes will depend on whether there is a history of diabetes in your family.

Often diabetes disappears after the birth of the baby. However, it is a sign that you have latent diabetes and it would be a good idea to keep a check on your diet and weight.

TOXAEMIA

When a woman's blood pressure is up the whole day (not just when she visits the clinic), when her urine test shows that there is albumin in the urine and when she is retaining fluids so that her fingers, ankles and possibly her face is swollen, she has toxaemia. A woman with toxaemia might also experience sudden weight gain. In severe toxaemia the placenta—which nourishes the baby, provides it with oxygen and helps excrete its waste products—will not be able to function well, so that there is a risk to the baby. In such cases, labour will be induced so that the baby is born while the placenta is still functioning well (see p. 36).

VERY HIGH BLOOD PRESSURE

In the last 3 months of pregnancy, when a woman's blood pressure is checked during an antenatal visit and is found to be high, say, 140/90 or more, the doctor will try and treat the high blood pressure so that the pregnancy can be maintained to allow adequate growth and maturity of the fetus, so that it will be able to survive at birth. Often rest might control the blood pressure. If required, sedation may be given to control it. If these measures are inadequate, labour may be induced (see p. 57).

WHEN THE WATER BAG BURSTS

When the water bag bursts in a great gush, and contractions do not start spontaneously, induction is set up to deliver the baby within 24 hours. This is what hospital protocol dictates. The reason this protocol is in place is because of the fear that beyond 24 hours the risk of infection sets in. Interestingly, the risk of infection rises with each internal examination. In midwifery units this fact is recognized and a mother is not induced, nor given repeated internal examinations. They simply check her temperature, a rise in it would indicate infection.

In a hospital setting there is no harm if you wait for 4 to 5 hours or longer after the bursting of the bag before the drip is fixed. It is possible that, as you wait, the contractions may start on their own. Contractions that start spontaneously are gentler and less intense than those induced by the drip.

PROLONGED LABOUR

When labour lasts for many hours without progress, say, approximately 12 to 18 hours or more, induction could be used to speed up the progress of labour.

RHESUS-NEGATIVE

If you are rhesus-negative and there is a possibility that your baby is going to need blood transfusion at birth, labour may be induced so that your baby will be born at a time when laboratory facilities, the paediatrician and other staff will be available (see pg. 37, 38). However, this danger today is almost non-existent, since an injection of anti-D immunoglobulin is given to the mother in the antenatal period as a preventive.

In case the mother has not received this injection in the antenatal period, and after any miscarriage or abortion that she may have had, she will need to deliver in a well-equipped hospital.

11

BIRTH

STRAIGHTFORWARD UNCOMPLICATED BIRTH comprises 3 distinct stages. In the 1st stage of labour the mouth of the womb opens up and dilates to make way for the baby's head to pass through. In the 2nd stage of labour the baby passes through the vagina and is born. In the 3rd stage of labour, the placenta is delivered, having completed its function of nourishing the baby.

THE FIRST STAGE OF LABOUR

The 1st stage is the longest—about 18 hours with a little plus or minus. The 2nd stage could be from one hour to two hours and the 3rd stage could take about 10 minutes to 40 minutes. In the first delivery, the 1st stage is usually longer than in subsequent births.

In the 1st stage, the lips of the womb or cervix thin out and stretch apart over the baby's head, while the body of the uterus shrinks on the baby and pushes it towards the cervix. This is what happens during the contraction or pain of labour. Sometimes, before contractions are felt, a harmless, thick mucus discharge may be noticed. On the other hand, a water leak may announce the approach of labour (see p. 69).

When you go to the hospital, your husband or relative will be given certain forms to be filled up, while you will be taken to a room where you will be told to change into a hospital gown. Then your pubic hair will be shaved. It will be followed by an enema. An enema is a process whereby a tube is inserted in the anus and a fluid flushes the bowels thoroughly. This avoids the passing of stool during birth. Often, after an enema, contractions become stronger. Remember, an empty rectum and an empty bladder will aid the progress of labour, so in labour pass stool whenever you desire to and keep drinking fluids and pass urine every 60 to 90 minutes. A full bladder can cause discomfort and pain and inhibit uterine contractions. Later it can lead to diminished bladder tone and infection. Do not limit your fluid intake. You will specially get thirsty if you perspire a lot.

After the enema, your husband or relative will be permitted to join you, and can be with you until when you are ready for birth, and taken into the delivery room. If you have booked in a big hospital, you may not be permitted to have your husband or relative with you.

During labour your blood pressure could be taken now and then. The nurse would also take your pulse and temperature, and listen to the baby's heartbeat. The position of the baby may be ascertained by palpitating/touching your abdomen. An internal examination could also be carried out to check how many centimetres the cervix has dilated. A note would be made of whether the membranes have ruptured and whether there is any bleeding. You will be asked when and what you ate last and whether you have taken any medication.

Sometimes labour can begin with gentle contractions, and build up to stronger contractions as time goes by. Between contractions, you must make an effort to practise quick relaxation. If labour starts during the day, move about the house at leisure. If labour starts in the evening or night, try and get some sleep. Do not tire yourself out by being physically overactive. Conserve your energy for the other half of labour, but do try and remain upright. When you are upright, the pressure of the baby's head on the cervix will stimulate your uterus to contract. If you lie down for a while, remember lying on your side is better than lying on your back, since it relieves pressure on the vena cava, and the aorta, two major blood vessels carrying blood to and from the heart, so that the oxygen content of your blood is enhanced, much to your and the baby's advantage.

You will find further details on how you can remain upright and when not to remain upright in the chapter *Labour Time*.

Labour can be handled quite comfortably with breathing, various positions and relaxation techniques. However, there are some drugs that are used for pain relief in labour. Their use will depend on the discretion of your obstetrician. You may or may not need them during labour.

Drugs, analgesics and anesthetics are sometimes administered, although they are often unnecessary and can have harmful side-effects. Refrain from asking for them. Family members accompanying the woman in labour should avoid becoming unnecessarily anxious, constantly requesting the doctor to do something. Labour will take its own time.

Some women may have an unnatural or difficult birth. Sometimes complications arise in labour. However, in some cases risk factors are already present, for instance, a woman with a previous stillbirth/with a kidney problem/uncontrollable diabetes/uncontrollable high blood pressure or risk factors exclusive to the mother. In such cases a good public hospital, or a well-equipped private hospital, is a good choice.

A big public hospital generally has a highly experienced and qualified staff, blood bank facilities, a paediatric unit to take care of the newborn. Public hospitals also would have fewer commercial pressures.

SECOND STAGE OF LABOUR

The 2nd stage of labour is recognized by strong contractions coming every 1 to 2 minutes and lasting a whole minute. After a while the contractions will slow down. Typical of this stage is also the desire on your part to bear down and push the baby out. Some women feel nauseous at this stage of labour. The 2nd stage of labour begins when the cervix has dilated to its full 10 cm and ends with the delivery of the baby. At this stage you are taken into the delivery room and made to lie down on your back with legs bent at the knees and feet resting flat on the bed. Alternatively, you will be made to lie down on your back and your legs will be supported by a set of stirrups. The stirrup would support the back of your bent knee and ankles, as your legs are supported individually on either side.

PREPARED CHILDBIRTH

If labour progresses without drugs, while a woman uses prepared childbirth techniques or naturally handles labour in a relaxed way, the body produces endorphin hormones. Endorphins are natural painkillers and are secreted by the body during hard physical exercise and labour.

Some prepared childbirth methods concentrate only on psychologically training a woman for birth, while other methods equip a woman to deal with labour by using certain breathing rhythms, as explained in this book, in the chapter *Breathing and Relaxation for Labour*.

Prepared childbirth is ideal for a woman who would prefer to avoid medication in labour either completely or as long as possible. Just moving about in labour from one position to another, as one desires, reduces the discomfort of labour greatly. So does the practice of breathing and relaxation.

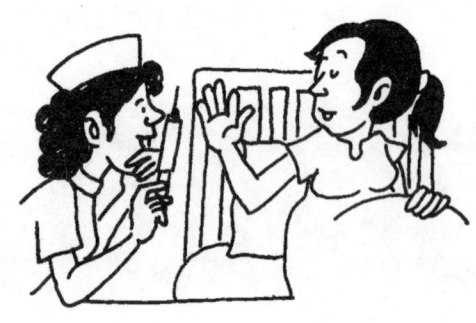

Painkillers are often freely offered and accepted in labour because in our civilized society nobody likes to lose emotional control. Women often say, 'I don't want to make an ass of myself.' It is not socially acceptable for a woman to make a show of her feelings in labour. She is expected to be a patient who lies down quietly in her bed, making as little noise as possible. Women often do not realize that they have another option.

It is best to avoid any kind of drug in labour, since whatever you inhale or receive intramuscularly, or through the drip while in labour, passes to the baby through the placenta in a matter of minutes. What you receive will be given to you in accordance with your body weight and it immediately passes to the baby who is only a fraction of your weight. So a drug that will make you sleepy or knock you out, will do the same, manifold, to the baby.

Most sedatives and painkillers given to the mother would depress her breathing and lower her blood pressure, doing the same to the baby. As a result the baby would be born sluggish, which may jeopardize the baby's respiration in the few precious moments after birth. Lack of oxygen at birth can have a serious effect on the child's brain, even if mild; it can affect its ability to learn in later years.

Drugs must be used with great caution, if the baby is premature or small, because the baby's liver will be immature and will find it difficult to break down the drugs and eliminate them from the baby's body. In labour, a drug, in order to be of use, should not be given in so large a dose that it results in dangerous side-effects. At the same time the dose should be large enough to give the desired effects, that is, the dose should not be too small and therefore ineffective.

The more medication a mother receives in labour, the longer and more difficult will be the baby's adjustment to life after birth. Medication can also affect breastfeeding negatively, especially in the first 5 days.

Most mammals like to have their babies in a quiet dark corner, where, left to themselves, they move about restlessly and deliver by themselves. People having pets may have noticed this kind of behaviour in dogs and cats. Human beings with their learned behaviour find it difficult to regress to such natural primitive behaviour.

A woman should learn to flow with her body and experience the birth of her baby as a basic function of her body. Each contraction should be considered an effort of her body to give birth to her baby. Handled positively and naturally, many women speak of the delight of feeling the baby's body slip through, of feeling a warmness and a wetness followed by the baby's cry. Whereas many drugged or anesthetized women may feel they missed out on it all.

Two obstetricians, Dr Dick Read and Dr Lamaze, taught women how to cope with labour. Dr Read stressed relaxation and understanding labour in order to remove fear. Dr Lamaze stressed teaching preconditioned breathing responses to women to use at the time of labour. Currently, Dr Michel Odent is teaching women how to regress to primitive consciousness in labour, by being given quiet and gentle support by birth attendants, while the labouring woman moves instinctively to find naturally comfortable positions. She is encouraged to forget what her culture has told her about labour, and to be in touch with her body.

In some big hospitals nowadays they have special beds on which mothers can birth the baby. These beds can get adjusted into an upright sitting-like position. They have flat fin-shaped supports for the mother's feet on either side. They also have at the bed level two handles that the mother can hold as she pushes the baby.

This is often referred to as the working stage of labour, for you have to work along with the uterine contractions to expel the baby and deliver it, by adding your efforts to physically push the baby out.

At this stage the folds in the vagina unfold to accommodate the baby's head. As the baby descends it could give a feeling of fullness in the rectum, which many women describe as a desire to pass stool. Finally the baby's head comes in contact with the perineum or the muscular outlet of the pelvis, which is stretched until the baby's head appears through it, just as your head would appear out of the top of a polo neck sweater when you are putting it on. The baby's head is normally delivered face down and the back of the head towards the ceiling. After the head is delivered, the baby's shoulders appear, followed quickly by the rest of its body. You may hear your baby's cry or whimper. The absence of a loud cry does not mean that something is wrong.

THIRD STAGE OF LABOUR

This stage begins with the birth of the baby and ends with the expulsion of the placenta, which peels away from the wall of the uterus and is delivered after the baby.

After the birth of the baby, the umbilical cord continues to pulsate and supply the baby with oxygen through the placenta, while simultaneously the baby's own breathing gets established. The cord is clamped a few inches away from the baby's navel and a few inches away from the clamp, it is incised or cut. A stump of the cord will be left on the baby's abdomen. After a few days the stump will dry up and fall off, leaving the baby's navel as a permanent mark of its past existence.

The baby is born with mucus or fluid in its nose, mouth and throat. Some of it is wiped away when the head is delivered. After birth the baby is kept head down to encourage further draining of the mucus. If the mucus seems to be interfering with the baby's first breath and there are chances of it being inhaled, it will be removed by a suction device. A little mucus remaining in the baby's lungs gets absorbed into the bloodstream when the baby's breathing is well established. At birth the baby's lungs are in a collapsed state like deflated balloons, stickily held together by mucus. The first breath fills them with air. The filling of the lungs with air causes blood to rush to them and the oxygen from the air is absorbed by the baby's bloodstream. When this happens the baby's blood circulation switches from receiving oxygen from the placenta to receiving oxygen from the baby's lungs.

The baby's heart starts to function. The artery that fed the baby's heart blood from the placenta stops functioning when the cord is incised, and the baby's heart begins to function independently.

The delivery of the placenta is not unpleasant or painful. The last few contractions cause the placenta to detach from the wall of the uterus and it is delivered through the birth canal. Sometimes an injection of syntometrine or syntocinon is given to make the uterus contract and hasten this stage. Sometimes the doctor tugs at the cord and at the same time the abdomen may be massaged to help free the placenta from the uterus. On the other hand, after 10 to 15 minutes of the birth, uterine contractions spontaneously start again. They take another 10 to 15 minutes to become strong enough to separate the placenta from the uterine wall and expel it.

The doctor checks the placenta to see that it has come out whole. Bits of it left inside can create problems later, of heavy bleeding and passing of clots.

THE BABY AT BIRTH

At birth a baby looks wet with plastered down hair. The body is covered with a cheesy substance called vernix which gives waterproof protection to the baby in the uterus. The baby might also be streaked with a little blood. At first the baby may look blue, but will change to a pink shade as its circulation gets established. At first the baby breathes around 110 breaths per minute and may cough and splutter or gasp.

Occasionally the baby's head might be a little oddly shaped as a result of its moulding during birth. The baby's breast may also be enlarged in either sex. A male baby's testes may seem blue and enlarged. A female baby's labia may be red and swollen. The baby may be covered with fine hair. After a few days the oddities of appearance will disappear.

Many babies have a bluish mark just above their buttocks. This fades with time in a few years.

VAGINAL BIRTH AFTER A CAESAREAN SECTION (VBAC)

THERE IS A common belief that if the first child was born by Caesarean section, the second delivery will also have to be by caesarean section.

This belief took root in about 1916 when Dr Edwin B. Craigin said, 'Once a Caesarean, always a Caesarean.' This statement of his has become medical dogma, and everyone has forgotten the medical conditions prevalent at the time when this statement was made.

Dr Craigin said this because around 1916, women laboured for many hours before a caesarean was considered. Caesareans were done with great fear and alarm because in those days, anesthesia techniques were not refined, and there were no antibiotics or blood banks. Unsterile conditions led to maternal and fetal mortality and morbidity.

In other words Caesareans were done only as a last resort. It was presumed therefore that if a woman had had a Caesarean section it must have been due to an obstruction in her birth passage since prolonged labour had not produced a child.

Craigin himself was very open-minded. He reported a case when his patient delivered vaginally three times after a Caesarean section. If a Caesarean is done for a non-recurring factor like the baby's heart going into distress or an unfavourable presentation of the baby at birth, a normal delivery can be attempted the next time.

According to N.K. Allahbadia, 'Vaginal Delivery following Cesarean Section', American Journal of Obstetrics & Gynecology, 85 (15 January 1963), No. 2: 'Once a Cesarean is NOT always a Cesarean!' According to him 97% rate of Vaginal Birth after Caesarean (VBAC) is possible.

In 1975 Nancy W. Cohen coined the term VBAC (pronounced we-back) and it began to be widely used.

In the 1980s the American College of Obstetricians and Gynecologists (ACOG) decreed that 'an attempt at vaginal delivery after cesarean childbirth appears to be an acceptable option.' The specific data used by the committee suggested 'that the risk of maternal mortality from uterine rupture is almost non existent, and the risk of prenatal death is relatively small'.

THE CAESAREAN SCAR OR INCISION

The incisions are actually two in number. One is the abdominal incision and the other is the incision on the uterus. Sometimes a woman may have a vertical incision on her abdomen, from her navel down to the pubic hairline, but the cut on her uterus may be on the lower part of her uterus and may be a horizontal cut. However, mostly the abdominal and the uterine cut are in the same direction.

The most commonly used uterine incision is in the lower segment of the uterus and is horizontal or transverse, that is, it looks like a dash; or a lying down line. The incision is made just above the mother's pubic hair, on her lower abdomen.

There are many advantages to the horizontal scar. Since it is done on the lower segment of the uterus, the area is not richly endowed with blood vessels, so massive haemorrhage is extremely rare. Repair is easier. Discomfort to the mother is less. Due to a low presence of muscle fibres in the lower segment of the uterus it does not participate very vigorously in the process of labour, and can therefore be depended upon in subsequent labour.

It was Dr Kerr who perfected the technique of the scar in the lower segment of the uterus. He worked on it in order to protect women and babies from the inherent risks that go with Caesarean sections. He urged his colleagues to use it, and then think of normal deliveries for subsequent labour.

Unfortunately, it is the perfection of this scar that has perpetuated the casual and repeated performance of Caesarean sections. In the rare event of a medical emergency today, we have tremendous back-up available to us from complete ante natal care to sophisticated anesthetics and suturing techniques, antibiotics, blood banks, etc.

This is very different from the early 1900s when the uterine incision often extended to the top segment of the uterus. The conditions for surgery were primitive and maternal mortality associated with Caesarean section was 10%. If several vaginal exams were done it could rise to 30%. Sometimes, in a woman with a previous Caesarean, if they delivered the baby two weeks early to prevent scar rupture, they ended up delivering premature babies that did not survive.

Nita, whose first-born was 4 years old, was expecting her second child in middle-February 2011. On checking her scar with ultrasound they said she should have a C-Sec because her scar, on 15 January 2011 was 1.66 mm when it should have been 3 mm (it was 4.4 mm in early December 2010, and 3 mm on 1 January 2011).

However, she successfully delivered vaginally in early February. When performing an ultrasound on her, they would press on the scar and ask if it hurt. Fortunately, it never hurt on her scar.

It is interesting to know that pain on the scar is often considered a sign of potential rupture of the uterus. However, most ruptures are not accompanied by pain or tenderness.

According to a report by Meehan and others in British Medical Journal 2

(1972): 740, 'many patients with a history of Caesarean section will complain of tenderness over the lower abdomen in late pregnancy or during labour, but when a Caesarean is performed, or after the baby is born vaginally, the scar is intact; many labours are halted because of complaints of pain over the lower uterine segment, although pain is quite notorious for its inaccuracy as a diagnostic tool!'

According to Dr Odent, ultrasound measurements of the uterine scar are not accurate. The general rule is to decide during the first stage of labour. If the first stage is straightforward it means that the vaginal route is possible. If there is failure to progress it is better not to hesitate to do another C-section.

One may ask, if there is a problem with the scar, what are the signs a mother should be alert to?

SIGNS OF SCAR RUPTURE

According to Dr Odent if there is a problem with the scar (it occurs in 0.5% of VBAC trials) there is a failure to progress with poor quality contractions. A terrible pain persisting between the contractions would be another kind of alert.

The book *Silent Knife*, by Cohen & Ester says: 'Symptoms of uterine seperation may include all, some, or none of the following: abdominal pain, vaginal bleeding, shock, swelling over the lower segment, a rise in pulse followed by a drop in blood pressure, fever, or a board-like uterus which does not contract. In 173 labors that we have followed, none of these has been a problem.' A woman has a better than 99.5% chance of no problem with the scar. A positive attitude will help.

An interesting fact is that no uterus is immune to rupture. A normal non-Caesarean sectioned uterus can also rupture at a point of least resistance and most powerful contractions.

It can happen as a result of injection or medicines that induce the uterus to contract. It can happen from carelessness e.g. a rupture occurred when a stitch used on the mouth of the uterus was not removed before labour started. It can happen if the uterus was perforated during the performance of an abortion, or during insertion of an intra uterine contraceptive device.

A study by Golan in 1980 (in Obstetrics & Gynecology 56, November 1980:540) reported 93 cases of uterine rupture during a 5 year period.

Total number of uterine rupture 93		Maternal Mortality
Rupture in normal uterus	61	9
Rupture in women with previous Caesarean scar	32	0
Total	93	9

In the possibility of the uterine scar giving way, the incision generally opens neatly and gently like a zipper. In *Silent Knife* Cohen and Ester say, 'We found no reports of maternal death associated with the lower segment incision in all the studies we surveyed; the incidence of fetal death associated with vaginal birth after caesarean (VBAC) is agreed to be less than that with elective repeat Caesarean even by most reluctant VBAC skeptics.'

The uterine scar heals, like other scars in our body. Specially if the cut is neatly stitched back together, sometimes there is no trace of the former incision.

In *Williams Obstetrics*, (Pritchard & Mac Donald In 41, Chapter 2) Williams writes, based on his observations and inspections, 'the site of the previous operation may not be recognizable by gross examination or even microscopic study!'

WHEN THERE IS A RUPTURE

According to Douglas, etc., in the American Journal Obstetrics & Gynecology (August 1963), 'Emergency during labor for VBAC are rarely more urgent than any other situation encountered in obstetrics. He noted that in 3,000 such Caesarean women, there had never been an emergency as a result of rupture of the lower uterine segment, and that *no fetal losses due to rupture or that mode of delivery should be expected.*

The word rupture generally creates panic. People think of bursting, exploding blood vessels, heavy bleeding and a medical emergency.

LAYERED HEALING OF THE UTERINE SCAR
(LIKE A GAP WITHIN THE CRUST OF A VEGETABLE PATTY!)

According to Case et al, in Journal Obstetrics & Gynecology (British Commonwealth, March 1971), at the time of a repeat Caesarean, most obstetricians have seen a hole in the old uterine scar. This opening is called a 'window.' It occurs with some frequency and is considered to be a result of healing. It is not a rupture. A window shows no recent tearing of tissue.

This 'window' is not a tearing of uterine muscle due to labour. It is a result of the healing of an old scar. Therefore it is not of any consequence. It does not require urgent medical attention.

However, only a few of the studies differentiate between windows and rupture, or between complete and incomplete rupture. In most studies, windows are recorded as rupture and included in rupture statistics, *even though they are of no serious consequence!*

DO I HAVE A CHOICE?

MOST PEOPLE THINK they have to passively accept 'treatment' given to them. They feel that they have no choice in the matter.

The physician or doctor has several options on how to treat a patient. In order that he is guided, the Hippocratic Oath is supposed to provide direction. Hippocrates (460-377 BC) is considered to be the father of allopathic medicine.

Since he lived a very long while ago, the oath he had written for physicians has been restated many a time with an effort to keep in mind the changing circumstances and yet retain the ethical principles.

In some medical institutions it is forgotten, whereas in other medical colleges a newer version of it is in place.

The original Hippocratic Oath swears upon gods and goddesses that the oath will be upheld. That the physician's teacher will be as dear as parents. That, in the course of practice, no deadly medicine will be dispensed. That the physician will enter a house to benefit the sick and abstain from mischief and corruption, will refrain from seduction, keep the secrets of the patients, and live a life of respect.

Amendments to the oath are as follows:

In 1948 The World Medical Association, Geneva, added, 'I will not permit considerations of religion, nationality, race, party, politics, or social standing to intervene between my duty and my patient... I will not use my medical knowledge contrary to the laws of humanity'.

This change was made after the Nazi experiments to create a super race.

Physicians for Compassionate Care added: 'I will treat the sick according to my best ability and judgement, always striving to do no harm.'

Some of the lines of the Hippocratic Oath taken at Tufts University, Australia are:

'I will remember that there is art to medicine as well as science, and that warmth, sympathy, and understanding may outweigh the surgeon's knife or chemist's drug.'

'I will remember that I do not treat a fever chart, a cancerous growth, but a sick human being, whose illness may affect the person's family and economic stability.'

The oath has provided the basis for ethical medical practice and patient welfare for the past 2,500 years. However, in modern-day medicine the struggle continues to retain its relevance.

One off-shoot of this struggle is 'Choosing Wisely', an initiative of the

ABIM Foundation, Philadelphia, USA, 2013.

The mission of the ABIM Foundation is to advance medical professionalism to improve the health care system. This is done by collaborating with physicians and physician leaders, medical trainees, health care delivery systems, payers, policy makers, consumer organizations and patients to foster a shared understanding of professionalism in practice.

Choosing Wisely aims to promote conversations between physicians and patients by helping patients to choose care that is:

- Supported by evidence
- Not duplicative of other tests or procedures already received
- Free from harm
- Truly necessary

Many experts agree that the current way health care is delivered in the US contains too much wastage—with some stating that as much as 30% of care delivered is duplicative or unnecessary and may not improve people's health.

Choosing Wisely has identified different specialities in medicine (Obstetrics, Cardiology, Rheumatology, Allergy, etc) and created a list of five points in each speciality. The list is titled 'Five things Physicians and Patients should question.' The five things are based on evidence as to what is the most appropriate care an individual can receive, based on their individual situation.

Let us look at the five things physicians and patients should question according to the list prepared by the American College of Obstetricians and Gynecologists:-

1. Don't schedule elective, non-medically indicated inductions of labour or Caesarean deliveries before 39 weeks 0 days gestational age.

Delivery prior to 39 weeks 0 days has been shown to be associated with an increased risk of learning disabilities and a potential increase in morbidity and mortality. There are clear medical indications for delivery prior to 39 weeks 0 days based on maternal and/or fetal conditions. A mature fetal lung test, in the absence of appropriate clinical criteria, is not an indication for delivery.

2. Don't schedule elective, non-medically indicated inductions of labour between 39 weeks 0 days and 41 weeks 0 days unless the cervix is deemed favourable.

Ideally, labour should start on its own initiative whenever possible. Higher Caesarean delivery rates result from induction of labour when the cervix is unfavourable. Health care practitioners should discuss the risks and benefits with their patients before considering induction of labour without medical indications.

The other three points are not relevant to childbirth, and therefore not mentioned.

For more information visit www.acog.org.

WHO Recommendations (Source: Lancet *(AQ:) 1985, 2:437)*

The World Health Organization (WHO) recognizes the importance of natural childbirth, and recommends that minimum technology be used in childbirth. In 1985, WHO held a conference on appropriate technology for birth. Over 50 participants specializing in obstetrics, paediatrics and other relevant professions came together in Fortaleza, Brazil. The participants unanimously adopted recommendations which WHO believes are relevant to the entire world. (*Lancet,* 1985, 2:437)

WHO recommends:

IT IS NOT RECOMMENDED THAT PREGNANT WOMEN BE PLACED IN A DORSAL LITHOTOMY POSITION DURING LABOUR AND DELIVERY. WALKING SHOULD BE ENCOURAGED DURING LABOUR AND EACH WOMAN MUST FREELY DECIDE WHICH POSITION TO ADOPT DURING DELIVERY.

In simple words, what this means is that women in labour should be allowed to adopt upright positions like walking, standing, sitting, kneeling, etc., rather than being made to lie down flat on their backs. Indeed, in labour, when a woman lies flat on her back, it is of disadvantage to her because of the following reasons.

Firstly, it results in the compression of a major blood vessel called the vena cava, which is positioned between the pregnant uterus and the mother's backbone. Compression of this blood vessel reduces the flow of blood to and from the heart, thus reducing the amount of oxygen available in the mother's body, to be used by both the mother and the baby. Therefore, if the mother does not lie flat on her back, the amount of oxygen available to mother and baby will be greater, so that both will be less likely to be distressed.

Secondly, when the mother lies flat on her back, her vagina is at an upward slant towards the front of her body. For the baby to be born, the uterus has to work harder, by shrinking more forcefully on the baby, to nudge it up the vagina. It is similar to climbing up a mountain. When the mother is upright, on the other hand, the baby has a downward descent, like going down a slide. This downward descent becomes speedier by virtue of the baby's body weight. In 1868 it was calculated that the weight of a full-term baby was enough to supply much of the force needed to expel it, provided the mother was upright. As we are aware, the force of gravity pulls things down in accordance to their weight. That is, a brick will fall quickly with a thud to the ground by virtue of its weight, whereas a feather will gently float to the ground because it is light in weight. An average Indian full-term baby weighs about three kilos, or six pounds. When the mother is upright, it is this weight of the baby that pulls the baby downward through the vagina.

It also puts pressure on the mouth of the womb, encouraging it to open.

Thirdly, as the baby slides down the mother's body to be born, it exits from the lower end of the mother's pelvic structure. Part of the lower circumference of the mother's pelvic structure comprises the tailbone. The tailbone is a free and flexible bone which very easily moves out of the way, giving the baby a few extra centimetres to be born, provided the mother is not in any way restricting its movement. Its movement can be free when the mother is in an upright position.

(See p. 70 for Precaution)

Interestingly, till modern obstetrics came about and birth went to the hospital, all the world over birth was always in an upright position. In Asia, women sat up or squatted during birth; in the West, birth-stools were used. Three factors contributed to this change:

(1) King Louis XIV of France wanted to watch his mistress give birth. He had her lie down at the time of birth and this made it fashionable to lie down at birth.
(2) Birth went from the home and the midwife to the hospital and the doctor.
(3) The use of forceps came about, which required the mother to lie down.

THE WELL-BEING OF THE NEW MOTHER MUST BE ENSURED THROUGH FREE ACCESS OF A CHOSEN MEMBER OF HER FAMILY DURING BIRTH AND THROUGHOUT THE POST-NATAL PERIOD. IN ADDITION, THE HEALTH TEAM MUST PROVIDE EMOTIONAL SUPPORT.

According to the Royal College of Midwives and the Royal College of Obstetricians and Gynaecologists, UK, the presence of a supportive companion in labour is one of the most effective forms of care in childbirth.

The Midwives Information and Research Service points out, 'ten randomised, controlled trials, which included over 3000 women, have examined the impact on a woman's labour, of having the continuous presence of a support person ... This person ... had received brief preparation on how to support women during labour.' The results are remarkably consistent, they show that continuous support is associated with: lower use of pharmacological anesthesia and fewer epidurals.

- fewer instrument deliveries (example, forceps.)
- fewer Caesarean sections.
- more five minute Apgar scores greater than seven. (That is, more babies were born alert, with a good supply of oxygen).

All these trials which looked at women's preferences found that continuous support is associated with:

- labour being better than expected.
- a more positive overall experience for the woman.
- There were no negative outcomes associated with 'support in labour'.

IMMEDIATE BREASTFEEDING SHOULD BE ENCOURAGED EVEN BEFORE THE MOTHER LEAVES THE DELIVERY ROOM.

The baby is alert at birth, so it is best to feed within 30 minutes of birth.

When the baby is born to a mother who has not received any drugs like pethidine, Calmpose, etc., in labour, it is born very alert. If such a baby is placed at the mother's breast, it will start suckling. This brings forth a gush of maternal love in the mother, who might until then be wondering about the odd appearance of her newborn. Hence, it is said to encourage bonding.

This happens because suckling at birth causes a release of oxytocin hormone in the mother. This hormone also causes the uterus to contract, the placenta to be expelled and haemorrhage to stop. The baby also gets drops of colostrum from the mother's breast, which is a precursor to breast milk. Colostrum provides the baby with immunity and protects it from allergies later in life. It also provides the baby with good gut health for the rest of its life. It is the first feed the baby gets for the first 4 to 5 days of his life after which time colostrum turns into milk.

Apart from the above advantages the baby learns to latch on properly to the breast for feeding and does not need to be coaxed and taught later when milk comes in.

The baby does not need glucose water or artificial milk/formula in the first day or two. The best is to breastfeed the baby only when it demands a feed (which initially can be after six hours or more, because colostrum has a high amount of fat) and to feed it nothing else. Artificial feeds fill the baby's stomach and prevent suckling at the breast.

Realizing the importance of this, there is an international effort called the Baby Friendly Hospital Initiative (BFHI). These hospitals as a matter of routine avoid over-medicating the mother and encourage breastfeeding at birth and afterwards.

If you want to breastfeed your baby at birth, you could speak to your doctor about your desire. This would include your desire to avoid sedatives being given to you in labour. If you feel shy or embarrazed, do not be so. Remember, for the doctor it is one of the ever so many deliveries. For you and your baby, however, it is a unique experience that will be etched in your memory for a lifetime.

OBSTETRIC CARE THAT CRITICIZES TECHNOLOGICAL BIRTH CARE AND RESPECTS THE EMOTIONAL, PSYCHOLOGICAL AND SOCIAL ASPECTS OF BIRTH SHOULD BE ENCOURAGED.

Using technology in birth stems from the belief that birth is a medicalised event of tremendous risk. According to Ros Claxton in *Birth Matters* (Unwin Paperbacks, 1986), 'the routine application of medical techniques that occurs in most hospitals creates more problems than it solves. Professor G.L. Kloosterman, the Dutch obstetrician, believes that 80-90 per cent of women are capable of normal deliveries without medical intervention'.

Somewhere along the line, people forget that birth is a normal biological event.

Most of the techniques used at birth have not undergone thorough testing. An interesting fact is that the fetal heart monitor, which is strapped onto the mother's abdomen and requires her to lie on her back, causes fetal distress. That is, it causes abnormal heartbeat of the baby, because, when lying on her back, the mother compresses a blood vessel. So this machine which was designed to identify fetal distress, is found to be actually causing it, if over-used.

It is interesting to know that, during, the Second World War, there was a tremendous strain on medical facilities and specialist care for pregnancy and birth nearly came to a stop. At this time, for some unexplainable reason, obstetric mortality rates (infant and mother death rates) fell to an unprecedented degree. This worldwide phenomenon seems to have no explanation. (Source: *Pursuing the Birth Machine*, Ace Graphics, 1994, by Dr M. Wagner, consultant to WHO on Women and Child Health.)

INFORMATION ON BIRTH PRACTICES IN DIFFERENT HOSPITALS, SUCH AS RATES OF CAESAREAN SECTION, SHOULD BE AVAILABLE TO THE PUBLIC.

This will help the public decide where they want to have their children delivered. They can choose a hospital where the percentage of Caesarean section is low, where the use of routine medications is not the norm, where breastfeeding is encouraged, where they will be allowed a labour companion, and so on.

THE INDUCTION OF LABOUR SHOULD BE RESERVED FOR SPECIFIC MEDICAL INDICATIONS. NO REGION SHOULD HAVE RATES OF INDUCED LABOUR HIGHER THAN 10%.

According to Wrigley (1962), it is 'questionable whether the oxytocin drip saved the life of a single baby and it is certain that its employment never made labour more normal or more comfortable for the patient'.

However, induction of labour would be medically required if the mother suffers from high blood pressure, diabetes, kidney problem, etc.

If induction of labour is over-used it can lead to the rupture of the uterus and a medical emergency.

Futher, as Sheila Kitzinger writes in her book, *Freedom and Choices in Childbirth*, 'Induced labours have disadvantages. They tend to be more painful, so induction starts a process in which powerful pain-killing drugs may have to be given. These in turn slow down labour and may lead to a forceps delivery. Induced labours are more likely than spontaneous labours to end in a Caesarean section'.

ARTIFICIAL EARLY RUPTURE OF MEMBRANES AS A ROUTINE PROCESS IS NOT JUSTIFIABLE.

Sometimes, doctors may burst the bag of water routinely. What this would do is speed up the birth process. To do this routinely is not recommended, it could lead to distress of the baby, infection in the mother and/or baby, cord prolapse etc.

The textbook *Common Obstetric Problems* by Ian Donald says, 'With very few exceptions, intact membranes mean an intact mother and an intact baby.'

DURING DELIVERY THE ADMINISTRATION OF ANALGESIC OR ANESTHETIC DRUGS (NOT SPECIFICALLY REQUIRED TO CORRECT OR PREVENT ANY COMPLICATION) SHOULD BE AVOIDED.

Drugs are not beneficial to the baby when the mother is pregnant, neither are they beneficial to the baby when the mother is in labour.

Drugs used in labour pass through the placenta and reach the baby's blood circulation, exerting a similar effect to that which is exerted on the mother. Since the baby receives the same dose as the mother, it becomes a massive overdose for the baby. If the mother recovers from the drug in two hours, the baby could take twenty hours to recover from its effect. After birth the baby may be given an antidote injection to the drug. Some drugs may remain in the baby's system and strain the baby's immature liver in breaking down and excreting the drug. This could lead to jaundice in the baby.

Apart from drugs, the discomfort of labour can be reduced in several ways. For instance, if the mother has a warm bath or is soaked in a tub of warm water. (Note: the temperature of the water in the tub should be body temperature, that is, 98.4° F.)

Also, moving about in labour and having a sympathetic caring companion would greatly reduce the 'pain' felt by a woman in labour.

Further, a positive attitude, coupled with conscious 'breathing' and relaxation techniques practised by the mother in labour will make labour comfortable for her. So will specific stroking and massaging techniques.

However, it is not a good feeling to go into a hospital with the thought that you and your partner are going to say 'no' to routine medication or procedures. It is better to discuss your choices in advance with your doctor. You could follow it up with a list of preferences stating your choices. The list of your preferences could be attached by your doctor to your case papers. This would be of great convenience to your doctor and to you. If the nursing home and/or staff is not willing to allow you your preferences and choices you could consider a change.

The following is an example of how a list of preferences could be:
1. You would like to have minimum of ultrasound.
2. You want a companion of your choice to be present with you during labour.
3. You wish to be able to move around in labour. (You will lie down for examination and if it is a case of a floating head and the water bag bursts.)
4. You do not need to have your water bag broken routinely.
5. You do not wish to have medical intervention until you are informed of its necessity.
6. You would like to hold your baby skin to skin, and breastfeed at birth, both in case of a normal delivery or a Caesarean section delivery. (See pp. 119). The baby is to be wiped and put on your chest soon after birth. Since the baby may take time to attach to the breast, the baby is to be left at the breast for about 30 minutes.
7. You would like to breastfeed the baby exclusively, and so you would not like the bottle of formula milk or glucose water to be given to the baby.
8. You would like to keep the baby with you in your room. It is called rooming-in of the baby.

9. In case your baby is put in special care after birth you would like to hold your baby skin to skin and give it expressed breast milk, or feed it directly.
10. You would like to attach a copy of your requests with your hospital notes.

GENTLE BIRTH

14

IN RECENT YEARS the limelight has shifted from the labouring mother to the labouring baby. At first all attention was focused on providing pain relief to the mother. Now, science has realized that the baby is not born deaf and insensitive to its environment as was previously believed. The baby is very sensitive to light, sound and touch. Just as the mother labours to give birth, the baby labours to be born, to wriggle itself out of the birth passage, to see the light of day.

Birth is also painful for the baby, how painful, one cannot say, since no one remembers the birth experience. Until labour begins, the baby is safe inside the warm water in the uterus. The baby does not have to breathe. Its body is supplied with oxygen through the umbilical cord. It is never hungry or thirsty. Nourishment reaches the baby through the cord. It is nurtured by the placenta and the umbilical cord and feels safe and familiar with its environment. Suddenly, the nurturing womb becomes hostile and begins to shrink on it, the space getting more cramped with each contraction. It gets expelled towards the opening in the mouth of the womb. From the womb it is propelled farther down towards the birth passage. Realizing the inevitable expulsive efforts of the womb, the baby also tries to struggle free in the direction of the expulsive forces. It joins in the struggle in the hope of setting itself free of these incomprehensible forces.

Finally comes freedom, or birth. And what does the baby encounter? In order to survive, it has to breathe, and quickly. For the cord supplying it with oxygen is cut immediately. Its lungs fill with air for the first time in its life, and it probably feels the passage of air searing in, and finally reach in its lungs to inflate them instantaneously like bicycle tyres. There is blinding light, which causes it to close its eyes. It gets held upside down and probably slapped, so that its cry can reassure birth attendants that all is well.

There are strange sounds or deafening noises. Its skin, used to the soft touch of warm water, experiences the rough feel of fabric. It gets laid on a cold, hard table. Tubes may be pushed into its nose/mouth right down to its lungs. Burning eye drops may be put in its eyes.

In other words, the trauma of labour is followed by the trauma of birth. Today, many psychologists feel that the trauma of birth can leave a permanent mark on the baby's psychology. Also, many obstetricians believe that the trauma of birth can be greatly reduced by giving a warmer welcome to the baby at birth.

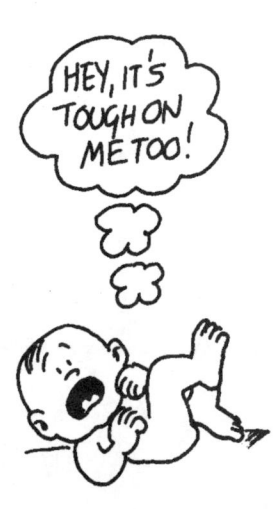

DR R.D. LAING

According to him, when the baby is born, the umbilical cord is wet and pulsating. It is full of blood which reaches the baby through it, from the placenta. As soon as the baby is born, the doctor clamps the cord and cuts it. It takes approximately 5 minutes for the baby's own blood circulation to establish. If the cord is not cut immediately, it gives the baby oxygen while this transition is being made. The blood vessels carrying blood from the cord seal off as the baby's own system of circulation takes over. So if the cord is cut after the newborn's own circulation has taken over, the newborn's adjustment to breathing and the world will be smoother and gentler.

DR FREDERICK LEBOYER

Dr Leboyer, a French obstetrician, feels that the baby's cry at birth is a cry of anguish from the pain it suffers. He believes the baby should be delivered in a gentle and loving environment of dim lights and hushed voices. The newborn baby should be lifted and placed face down on the mother's abdomen. The mother should gently massage the baby's back as it unfolds into the world. The cord should be cut after it has stopped pulsating, even though the baby would have been breathing on its own for some time.

Leboyer in his book, *Birth without Violence* (UK, 1975), says, 'Instead of howling as expected, each baby merely uttered two or three healthy cries and then contented itself with powerful breathing. So that in the silence that followed, what each woman heard was the very absence of her baby's cry. Her eyes soon betrayed first surprise and then alarm, darting questioningly from one of us to the next.

'Why isn't my baby crying?' They seemed positively aggrieved. The surprise, the regret, the accusation in those questions dumbfounded us. We had not realized how deeply ingrained is the assumption that the newborn child must cry, how profound is the unconscious acceptance that birth and suffering are one.

'To be fair, we must admit that a newborn baby who begins gurgling happily after just a cry or two, who yawns and stretches, who enters life the way we awake from a restful sleep—is something of a surprise.

'When a child comes into the world, it must undoubtedly cry. But it need not weep.'

Once the cord is cut, Dr Leboyer believes the baby should be lowered gently in a small tub or basin of warm water. The baby will feel the warm lightness of moving in water, just as when it was safe and warm in the water bag, in the mother's womb.

DR MICHEL ODENT

Dr Odent has been greatly influenced by Dr Leboyer's teachings.

However, while Dr Leboyer concentrates on the baby, Dr Odent also takes into account the woman in labour. He believes that a woman should be trained to accept labour as a very natural process of her body, and that she should regress to her primitive consciousness to be in touch with her body while it is accomplishing a very basic function. Women should be taught various upright positions they can adopt in labour. In labour a woman should do whatever she wants to. She can go through labour as she likes.

If she wants to scream, she screams. If she wants to sit she sits, walks if she wants. The room where she delivers has no menacing stainless steel equipment exposed. It is done up in warm shades of orange and brown. The room is softly lit and comfortable. It could have a low platform, cushions and birthing chair. A woman is told to remain upright in labour and to give birth in a squatting position, just as advocated by the traditional Indian *dais* (midwives).

Dr Odent feels this is especially useful in delivering breech babies, or babies being born feet first. When a mother is squatting at birth, a breech baby gets born much faster, so that the danger of the baby breathing in mucus before the head is delivered is greatly reduced.

Dr Odent also has a small pool of warm water in which a woman in labour can sit. The warm water relaxes a woman's tense muscles and eases contractions. Babies are sometimes born in the pool of warm water when the mother does not desire to leave the pool. The baby emerges into the water while it is still getting oxygen from the umbilical cord. It transfers from the watery medium of the womb to the watery medium of the pool. It breathes when it is lifted out of the water of the pool.

Dr Odent's uniqueness lies in his belief that each woman possesses an instinctive ability to give birth naturally. This ability is held suspect by modern obstetric practice, which concentrates on skills to control labour. Dr Odent witnesses each birth as it occurs and does not intervene in any way. He does not use pain-killing drugs, synthetic hormones, epidurals or forceps. He believes that without any medical intervention the body releases complex neurohormones. It is on the natural balance of these hormones that spontaneous labour depends.

Dr Odent in his book, *Birth Reborn* (UK, 1986), says, 'It has also become more and more obvious that endorphins play an important role in the complex hormonal equilibrium that makes a spontaneous delivery possible. Neurohormones with morphine like functions, these 'endogenous opiates', act as natural pain-killers, not only protecting against pain but also suppressing anxiety and inducing a general feeling of wellbeing. High levels of endorphins may, for example, induce so called alpha brain waves that are associated with states of serenity or beautitude. It is almost as if people have always sensed the presence of this natural capacity for wellbeing and sought ways to trigger it. Running, for example, raises our endorphin levels; prayer, meditation, yoga and acupuncture may do the same.'

After the baby is born, it is placed on its stomach, on a soft towel between the mother's legs. The baby's head is turned to a side so that if the baby has some liquid in the mouth, gravity helps to drain it out and prevent it from entering the baby's lungs. The baby lies like this until it lets out a cry and takes some deep breaths, coughs, sneezes and shows good body tone. The room is heated to a comfortable temperature or the baby is covered with a blanket. Then the baby is scooped up by the mother in her arms while it is still linked to her body by the cord. In the first half hour or so after birth, mother and baby get to know each other. The cord is cut unhurriedly after this first contact has been made.

(Cesarean Section Rates)	
Dr Odent	6 to 7%
U.S.A.	19%
U.K.	13%
France	15%

In France perinatal mortality rates (i.e. death immediately before or after birth) in the last 8 years have dropped from 20 per 1,000 to 10 per 1,000. Dr Leboyer is said to have greatly contributed to this.
(These statistics are from the 1980s.)

Source: Birth Reborn *by Dr M. Odent (p.101)*

Although Dr Leboyer and Dr Odent strongly believe in gentle birth, they are backed up by a full medical team should emergencies occur. They know how to look out for maternal or fetal distress, should it occur, and how to take care of it. Dr Leboyer points out that mother and child should never be allowed to go short on oxygen. Dr Odent performs Caesarean sections when they are necessary. Interestingly, their Caesarean section rate and their rate of babies dying are lower than the average.

BREASTFEEDING

WHY SHOULD I BREASTFEED?

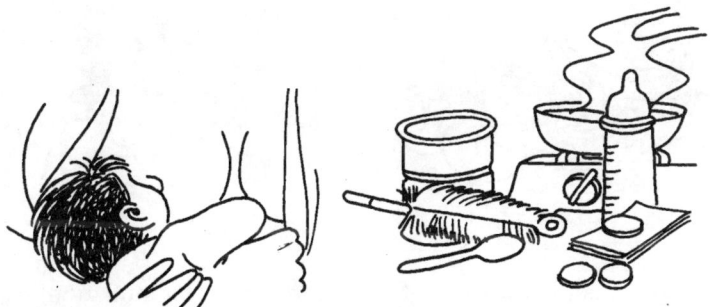

All you need is a mom and a baby! No other paraphernalia is required. Breast milk is nutritionally balanced and easily available. It prevents disease and promotes health in the baby. Best of all, it costs nothing, and is produced according to consumer demand! If a mother has twins she will produce milk for two babies! It comes sterilized, and at the right temperature.

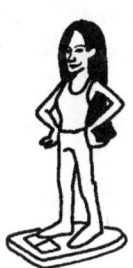
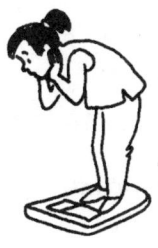

Breastfeeding helps the mother lose weight, and encourages her uterus to contract to its normal size and position. The incidence of breast and ovarian cancer, anaemia and osteoporosis tends to be lower in women who have breastfed.

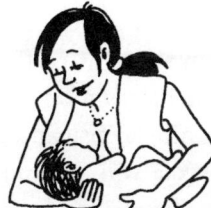
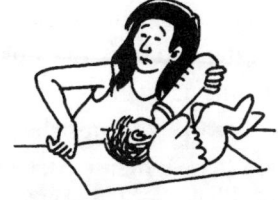

Breastfeeding helps babies feel loved and secure. It encourages bonding.

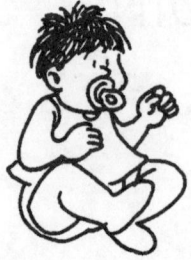 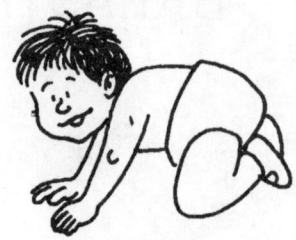

Breastfed babies are thinner but more active and smarter

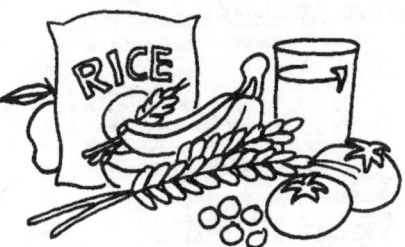 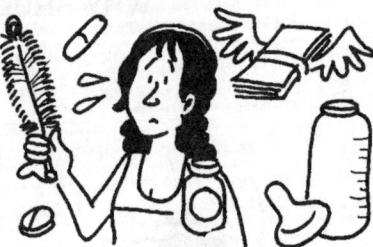

The mother and the whole family can get better nutrition, instead of enormous amounts of money and energy being spent on bottle feeding.

Breast milk is best for the proper growth of the baby. It also helps the baby's brain development.

In pregnancy, fat is deposited in the mother's body to be used during feeding. Mother's milk has fat and lactose (carbohydrate) in it; so you lose weight faster than a woman who is bottlefeeding.

Breast milk also protects the baby from allergies, and from disease. Since breast milk is always pure, breastfed babies have fewer episodes of diarrhoea.

DOES BREASTFEEDING MAKE BREASTS SAG?

You may hear 'Breastfeeding makes your breast sag.' Unfortunately, breasts sag all by themselves as you age. Whether you breastfeed or not makes no difference—even women who never get pregnant must eventually face the reality of sagging of breasts when they grow older. If you wear a good supportive bra while feeding, breastfeeding need not cause the breasts to sag.

HOW DOES THE BABY FEED?

The baby's gums press on the areola, that is, the dark area behind the nipple. The nipple gets extended back towards the baby's gullet, and the baby's tongue milks it, by pressing it against the roof of the baby's mouth or palate.

If the baby incorrectly munches on the nipple instead of the areola, it will hurt the mother. A major part of the areola will continue to be visible both above and below, and the baby will be dissatisfied because not much milk will come.

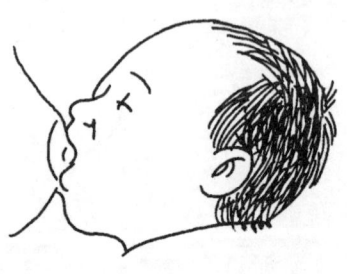

WRONG

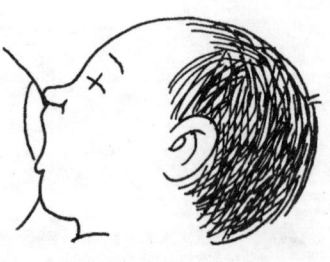

RIGHT

On the other hand, when the baby is feeding correctly, more of the dark area of the mother's breast shows above the baby's upper lip and less under the baby's lower lip.

Since the baby has to munch for each sip of milk, its jaw development improves. Also, it makes it possible for the baby to pause in between, just to breathe or look around.

As opposed to this, a bottle-fed baby suffers a respiratory load as he gets a continuous flow of milk through the bottle's nipple. It also makes the baby tend to overeat. So the seeds of becoming overweight are sown right at the start.

HOW TO FEED

When the baby latches onto the breast to feed, and it hurts, it is possible the baby has not latched on properly. If the baby's gums press on the nipple it will hurt. If the baby's gums correctly press on the dark area behind the nipple, the baby's sucking will not cause any discomfort. Correct sucking releases the flow of milk, and causes relief to the mother, especially if the breasts are hard and sensitive from being overfull. The release of milk is accompanied by a tingling sensation of the breasts. Further, the muscle below the baby's ears move as the baby sucks and swallows.

If the baby's sucking hurts, in order to correct the latching, insert a finger in the baby's mouth, between the gums, so that the baby's mouth opens and you can take the baby off the breast.

Position the baby sideways, so that the baby's tummy & the mother's tummy face each other. The baby's nose should be in line with the mother's nipple. The baby's mouth touches the breast below the nipple and the baby opens her mouth and sticks her tongue out. At that moment the mother can put the nipple into the baby's open mouth. This ensures the baby gets a good mouth full of breast. Therefore, a baby well latched, typically, has her mouth wide open.

COLOSTRUM

Feeding the colostrum (a clear fluid present in the breast for 3 to 4 days before milk comes in) helps to teach the baby how to suck, so that when the milk comes in, baby's sucking brings relief to the mother.

If the colostrum is not given to the baby, and instead sugared water or bottle milk is repeatedly fed, the baby will get used to getting a constant flow from the bottle's nipple without having to suck very much.

Colostrum is present in the breast after the sixth month of pregnancy and therefore even premature babies can benefit from it. It is full of immunities the mother has, so the baby does not catch infection easily. It is very high in fat and protein and acts like a laxative, encouraging the baby to pass its first stool and reduces jaundice in the baby. (see p. 124)

After a few days, when milk comes in, the breasts are painful and sensitive.

SIGNS THE BABY IS CORRECTLY LATCHED ON

The baby's chin touches the mother's breast

The lower lip curls outwards

More of the areola shows above the baby's upper lip and less under its lower lip.

The baby is held sideways by the mother in a straight line, so that the baby is tummy to tummy with her.

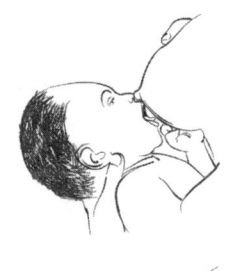
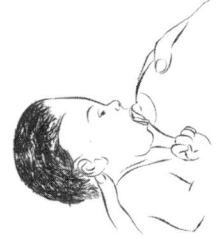
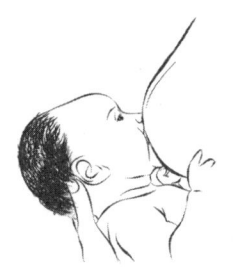
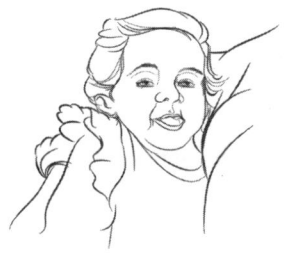

A baby who has had the colostrum will relieve this discomfort by sucking at the breast and emptying it. But a baby who has not sucked at the breast before will take time to learn and during this learning process cause considerable discomfort to the mother.

FAT-RICH HIND MILK

If the baby empties one breast entirely, it gets the fat rich Hind milk which makes the mother lose weight and the baby put on weight. This will also give the baby greater satisfaction after a feed. When a breast empties it gets smaller in size and lighter in weight. Also, feeding in this manner ensures the thorough emptying of both breasts.

If the baby is still hungry you could feed it from the other side briefly. Start the next feed from the side you fed briefly from.

When the baby has had enough she leaves the breast spontaneously, and will not be interested in feeding further. While feeding the baby may stop and restart several times. A feed may therefore sometimes stretch to 40 minutes or more. Sometimes it could be over in 30 minutes.

BREAST SIZE

The size of breasts in no way determines success or failure when feeding. Women with fairly small breasts can feed as efficiently as women with large breasts.

Sometimes large pendulous breasts can be a problem while breastfeeding, because the nipple is very low and the mother can't see it, when she wants to direct it to the mouth of the baby. In such cases it helps if the mother places her hand next to her chest under the breast and raises the breast slightly. Her hand should hold the breast in a 'U' shape with the thumb on one side and the four fingers on the other side of the breast.

During pregnancy you will put on weight on the breasts, and as pregnancy advances you will need a larger sized bra. The size could increase by two sizes, that is, a woman normally wearing size 34 could need size 38 as a feeding bra.

After the baby is born, when the milk comes into the breast after a few days, the breasts become big, heavy and uncomfortable. In the first 2 to 3 months, the breasts will remain fairly large. At times hardness and fullness may also be experienced when the baby skips a feed. If you are uncomfortable you can express your milk and it can be fed to the baby later. (see pg. 127)

At about 2 to 3 months many mothers feel that they are not making enough milk. This is because by 2 to 3 months the breasts will go back to their normal size and feel soft, just as they were before pregnancy.

This does not mean that you are no longer producing milk. You might still be feeding the baby, but by this time the supply and demand balance is just right, and no overproduction of milk, or overfilling of breasts takes place. Continue feeding the baby without tension. Drink lots of fluids and relax when you feed. Remember, the body will produce milk on demand.

That is, the more you feed the more milk you will make. So do not skip a feed in the hope of collecting more milk for the next feed.

When feeding goes on for many months, some women might find their breasts going smaller than before they became pregnant. It will take them time to put on the fat again and to regain their original size.

FEEDING BRAS

The breasts are fat tissue held in place by pectoral muscles. These are muscles that cover the front of the chest. In order to make sure the breasts do not sag, we need to strengthen the pectoral muscles. (See Bust Exercise in chapter, 'Some Simple Exercises'.) When breastfeeding you need to do the bust exercise only in the central position i.e. palms joined in front of the breast in a slanting position.

Wearing a bra supports the breasts, when a woman stands up against gravity. When a woman lies down the breasts can do without the support of the bra.

It is best that women do not wear a bra when sleeping.

Wearing a bra when sleeping can hamper circulation, cause restlessness and prevent the mother from getting a good night's sleep.

It may also cause hyper pigmentation, that is, dark spots, discolouration or uneven skin tone. It may also cause fungus since it provides a long period of a warm and moist environment for fungus to grow.

According to Sydney Ross Singer, medical anthropologist, breast cancer researcher and co-author of *Dressed to Kill: the Link between Breast Cancer and Bras*:

'Sleeping in a bra is the worst thing to do for the breasts. Bra-free women have about the same incidence of breast cancer as men, while the incidence rises the tighter and longer a bra is worn, to over 100 times higher for a 24/7 bra user compared to bra-free. The compression of the breast tissue by the bra, which is evident by seeing red marks or indentations in the skin from the bra, results in fluid and toxin accumulation, causing pain, cysts, and ultimately, cancer. To find out if your bra is harming your breasts, try going bra-free for one month and feel the difference.'

A GUIDE TO BUYING FEEDING BRAS

1. During pregnancy, if the bra fits well but is tight below the breast, you could buy some extra bra hooks called 'bra extensions' that fix an eye and hook to the existing eye and hook at the back of the bra, making it broader in circumference and therefore comfortable.
2. When breastfeeding, a feeding bra should be worn, so that the breasts do not sag with the extra weight. Due to the extra weight of the breasts, the bra should be well-fitted and made of cotton, since cotton does not stretch with the increase in size, and therefore gives better support. It also allows better absorbency and circulation of air, hence reducing chances of sore nipples.
3. The bra should not be too tight at the cup. It should not have bands at the top of the breasts that cut into the skin when the front cup or flap opens for feeding.
4. Wear underwire bras only when dressed for an outing, not all the time. Particularly not when sleeping. You could avoid underwires altogether.
5. Broad cotton straps over the shoulders will give better support and comfort.

BRA SIZE

Most women are wearing the wrong bra size. To find the proper measurements, start by wearing a non-padded, well-fitting bra.

Wrap the measuring tape snugly around your rib cage, just under the bust line. Be sure the measuring tape is parallel to the floor all around. This measurement—for instance, 38 inches—is your band size. If you measure between sizes, round off to the next number for a comfortable bra, and round off to the previous number for a snug-fitting bra. Keep in mind that when you are nursing your breasts will become larger. Rounding off a band size up is therefore recommended.

To find your cup measurement, bring the measuring tape around the fullest part of your breast. Wrap the tape loosely over the breast. Subtract the number of this second measurement from the band size, for example, if the measurement around your breast is 41 inches and your band size is 38 inches, the difference would be three inches. Accordingly your cup size would be C, the third alphabet (for 3 inches). Bra sizes can be A (for one-inch difference), B (for two-inch difference), etc. Bra sizes can go up to D, E, etc. (Read 'Breast Size' above.)

WEARING YOUR BRA

To put on your bra well, do so standing. Wear the bra and bend forward from your waist so that the breasts fall into the cup. Then hook your bra from the back. Check your nipple alignment, adjusting to make both centred in their respective cups.

FLAT NIPPLES

If your nipples do not project as nipples normally do, and appear flat or dimpled, they are called flat or inverted nipples. Being flat, your nipples may project when you are cold, sexually aroused or when feeding the baby. Flat nipples are no longer considered to be a problem. As the baby suckles, a nipple-like shape gets formed.

An inverted nipple is a nipple that does not project. It looks somewhat like a navel. Lack of projection of the nipple, when the baby sucks, could make the baby unable to grasp the nipple in its mouth when feeding.

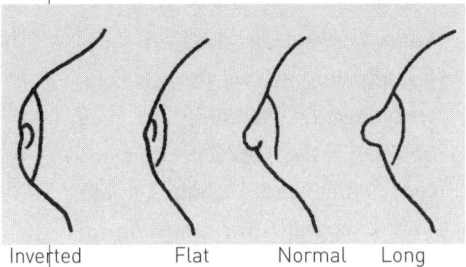

Inverted   Flat   Normal   Long

If you press on the areola and the nipple projects out, it should not be a problem to breastfeed. However, if the nipple retracts when you do that, then the syringe method is required during breastfeeding.

The syringe method was innovated by Dr Nirmala Kesaree, and is also referred to as the Nirmala Kesaree method.

To begin with, you need a 10 ml syringe. However, if the mother's breasts are very large you would require a 20 ml syringe.

Follow the steps as illustrated in the box, 8 to 10 minutes before a feed.

Apply the syringe on the areola and pull gently. This will cause the nipple to form. Maintain the position for 1 minute or 60 seconds. Then gently remove the syringe from the breast, taking about 20 seconds to do so.

Repeat 8 to 10 times before giving a feed, so that the areola will be projected at the time of the feed. That will make it easy for the baby to latch on.

Once the baby has latched on the nipple will remain projected for the rest of the feed. In a week or so, a 'permanent cure', that is, the projection of the nipple, comes about.

THE SYRINGE METHOD
(Nirmala Kesaree Method)

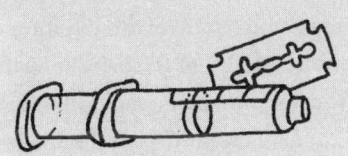

Remove plunger and cut the end on which the needle is inserted, with a cutter.

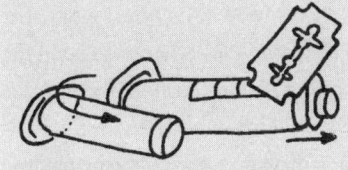

Insert the plunger from the cut side. Place the uncut side of the syringe on the areola and gently pull the plunger to help the nipple project.

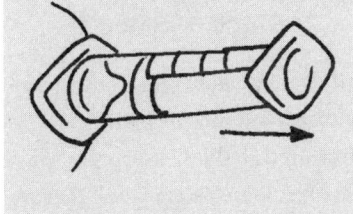

BREASTFEEDING AT BIRTH

If the baby is simply held in a relaxed manner, close to the mother's breast, within 30 minutes after birth, it will latch on to the mother's breast and start suckling. This is because babies are born with 3 reflexes:

- **Homing in reflex**: the baby moves towards the areola.
- **Rooting reflex**: the baby attaches itself to the mother's breast for feeding.
- **Sucking reflex**: the baby sucks at the breast.

When the baby is breastfed at birth, it immediately learns how to attach itself to the breast. It does not have to struggle to attach itself to the breast after the colostrum changes to milk, and the breast gets filled with milk. Besides, the colostrum (a clear liquid, present in the breast at birth) that it sucks will protect it from infections.

Breastfeeding at birth also promotes bonding. According to J.C. Pearce in his book *Magical Child* (1980), 'Bonding is stage specific. Nature has designed the bonds to be established in the hours immediately following birth…as is the case of learning to breathe, this is a critical period for bonding.'

Pearce further explains that when the mother breastfeeds her baby at birth she stimulates all the 5 senses of the baby, that is, touch, smell, sight (the baby can concentrate on a face 6 to 12 inches away from its own in the hour following birth), taste and hearing (since most mothers will 'talk' to the baby while feeding). This in turn stimulates the reticular formation of the brain (an area of the brain that receives messages from the 5 senses). It gives the baby better coordination between the brain and the 5 senses for the rest of its life.

When this happens, 'All adrenal steroid production has completely disappeared in a short time because the infant, in being returned to, and recognising the known, relaxes. He then remains in an alert and yet calm state of learning.'

ROOMING-IN

It is best for the mother to have her baby with her in her room and feed her on demand. Initially, before breast milk comes in, the colostrum, being heavy, will make the baby sleep long hours without demanding a feed. This gives the mother the rest she needs. Further, colostrum and breast milk give the baby immunity or protection from infection in the hospital and from visitors.

Each one of us has some bacteria or germs on our body. When the baby is next to the mother, it develops a bacterial flora that is similar to that of the mother. When the child is in the nursery, it can catch the bacterial flora of the nurse, who may be carrying some infection, or may not wash her hands before touching the baby. Plus, instead of getting the mother's immunity-rich, infection fighting colostrum, the baby may receive a bottle of milk, which will make it further susceptible to infection. It is therefore better for the baby to be with the mother. Glucose water or bottle milk may sometimes be given as a 'test feed'. If this test feed is aspirated into the baby's lungs, it can irritate them. Colostrum on the other hand, if aspirated into the lungs will not irritate, but simply get absorbed.

If you are expecting lots of guests, you could have the baby lie next to the mother on the bed and say the doctor has asked to keep the baby next to the mother. This is in fact an excellent thing to do with small babies, because they get the body heat of the mother, and the baby's own temperature control mechanism is not strained.

EXCLUSIVE BREASTFEEDING

Feeding only breast milk is recommended for 6 months. That is, no other milk, water or mashed foods needs to be given. The baby's digestive system is mature enough to digest a range of foods by 6 months. There is enough water in the breast milk for the baby. The mother will need to drink lots of water and eat nutritious food when she is feeding, since she is supplying nourishment and water to the baby.

The mother does not need to drink lots of milk to make milk. Apart

---

BABY-FRIENDLY HOSPITALS

Some hospitals are labelled baby-friendly hospitals if their policies encourage breastfeeding. In such hospitals, the resident doctors, consultant and labour room staff encourage breastfeeding of newborns, within half an hour in a normal delivery, and within 4 to 6 hours after a Caesarean delivery. Such hospitals also avoid the routine use of sedatives or analgesics which could lead to depression in the infant and interfere with the normal sucking reflex of the baby at birth. The health care staff in these hospitals should inform the mother of the advantages of exclusive breastfeeding and the disadvantages of artificial feeding. All newborns in such hospitals are routinely kept with the mother 24 hours a day. The baby's cot would therefore be in the mother's room, next to her bed. It is essential for baby-friendly hospitals to display their breastfeeding policy document in the antenatal clinic, maternity ward, special care nursery, etc.

STOOL OF BABIES

All babies pass the first stool within 24 hours of birth.
Breastfed babies normally pass very frequent watery stool, that are not wholly formed. Sometimes, with wind a bit of stool may be passed.
Bottlefed babies pass harder stool which may give rise to constipation.

from water she could have lots of other fluids like soups, fresh lime water, tender coconut water, etc.

CONSTANT FEEDING DEMAND

Some babies want to be constantly fed. According to one mother, within 10 to 15 minutes her baby would want to be fed again. When put to the breast again, however, she did not suck properly, so she gave her the bottle. On enquiry it was revealed that breastfeeding was the only time she held her baby. So what the baby was demanding was not a feed, but comfort sucking. If a baby seems to want constant feeding, it may not be asking for a nutritious feed, but comfort sucking. Abundant cuddling of the baby or strapping the baby onto the mother will reduce the baby's need to fake hunger, when what it actually wants is simply to be held close and feel secure.

Another time a baby may want constant suckling is when it experiences a growth spurt. When the baby grows, it needs more milk. Feeding more often increases milk supply. So, if suddenly the baby seems to want more feeding, just take a couple of days off. Stay in bed, eat well, and feed on demand. Once the supply is stepped up, the baby will stop demanding constant feeding.

The baby is also very sensitive to the mother's emotions and can get restless and cranky and want to feed constantly if the mother is emotionally disturbed.

LET DOWN REFLEX

When the milk is releasesd the mother experiences a tingling sensation in her breasts. That is the let down reflex.

This is a reflex that causes milk to be 'let down' and flow when the baby is feeding. If the mother is worried, stressed, extremely self-conscious, etc., it can interfere with the release of milk. It is therefore important that a breastfeeding mother is relaxed, so that her milk can flow freely. If tension prevents the let down reflex or interferes with it, a mother can buy from a Homeopathic medicines shop either Kali Phos 6X or Rescue Remedy, having them would help her to relax. She can have 2 hourly if very tense. Later, four times a day.

LEAKING BREASTS

As breastfeeding gets established, the breast may start leaking milk after a bath. Or when the mother feeds from one side, the other side may leak. Sometimes when it is time for the baby's feed, or when the mother lovingly thinks of the baby, the milk starts leaking. It is better not to wear water proof backed bra pads, since they cause the nipples to remain soggy and become sore. As the demand and supply settles down, leaking of breasts may reduce. You could fold some cotton in an absorbent men's cotton hanky and place inside the bra to avoid your clothes getting wet from leakage when you have company.

WHEN NOT TO BREASTFEED

Mothers suffering from tuberculosis, chronic nephritis (kidney trouble), or severe psychiatric disorders will be asked not to breastfeed; also mothers who have suffered from some malignant disease. Some patients of epilepsy may be discouraged from feeding if they are on a drug that can be excreted in breast milk.

Every day, after the sixth month

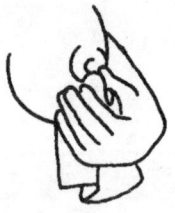

FEEDING WHEN ILL

Cold, flu, fevers should not require you to stop feeding. However, do let the doctor know that you are nursing the baby, when he prescribes you medicines. Feeding should continue as long as possible, so that the baby can get the maximum advantage of the immunities present in the mother's milk. An infected mother produces within her body antibodies to fight the infection she has. These are secreted in breast milk. They become available to the baby and protect him against infection.

MEDICATION

When feeding, antibiotics such as tetracycline and streptomycin, steroids and sulpha-containing drugs should be avoided.

Some laxatives may cause colic and diarrhoea in the baby. Anti-thyroid drugs may cause goitre. Anti-coagulants and large doses of aspirin can cause bleeding problems in the baby.

Sedatives or tranquilisers such as valium can cause drowsiness and feeding problems.

TO STOP FEEDING SUDDENLY

If, for some reason, you have to stop feeding abruptly, do it under your doctor's supervision. The doctor will give you a safe drug called bromocriptine that will dry up the milk. It is best to taper off breastfeeding gradually.

If the baby does not suckle at the breast and neither does the mother express milk, milk secretions will not stop. There is a substance which can reduce or inhibit milk production. If a lot of milk is left in the breast, the inhibitor stops cells from secreting milk anymore.

BREAST PREPARATION FOR FEEDING

From the sixth month of pregnancy onwards, certain breast preparation techniques have to be started, to ready the breasts and nipples for breastfeeding.

Although some schools of thought do not recommend breast preparation in pregnancy, our experience has been that it facilitates successful breastfeeding. We therefore highly recommend it.

Because of the manner in which the baby sucks, it is important to toughen the mother's nipples so that they do not give the mother discomfort when breastfeeding.

STEP 1

With a dry towel, clean the tip of the nipples. You may find dry scabs falling off. These scabs or flakes are formed when drops of colostrum get secreted unnoticed and dry at the tip of the nipple.

STEP 2

Hold both nipples like a cigarette, lightly between your forefinger and middle finger. Now draw the nipples in and out or forward and backward 50 times. If you press on the nipples with your fingers it can hurt, therefore remember to hold lightly.

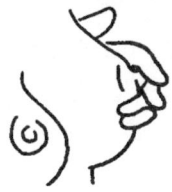

Each time the baby sucks, its gums press on the dark area behind the nipple, and the nipple gets extended way back towards the baby's throat, and the milk goes straight down the baby's gullet. By doing this action, you are acquainting the nipple with this action, which will be repeated frequently during a feed.

STEP 3

The third step in breast preparation requires you to hold the areola, the dark area behind the nipple, where the normal skin and the dark skin meet, between the forefinger and thumb, and press.

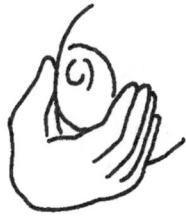

Move the fingers around and press all around the areola. You might notice a few drops of fluid appearing at the tip of the nipple. Don't worry if you do not notice any.

Wipe off the drops of fluid and lightly apply any natural, edible oil on the nipple and the areola. You can use coconut oil, ghee or groundnut oil, any other edible oil. Breast creams are best avoided. Also, scented oils or vitamins enriched oils are to be avoided.

The fluid that sometimes appears during this procedure is colostrum, a forerunner to breast milk. It is present in the breast from the sixth month of pregnancy onwards. It is highly useful when fed to infants and premature babies, since it has a large number of antibodies and therefore protects the baby from infection.

PRECAUTION

If you have premature contractions or bleeding or have been prone to either and are on medication to prevent them, do not breast prepare after the sixth month of pregnancy. Instead, do it 15 days before the estimated date of delivery.

WHEN FEEDING

The body has its own system of secreting lubrication from the Montgomery's tubercles (little prominences around the areola), to keep the nipple supple and oiled. However, during a bath when soap is used, it gets washed away, so women find rubbing oil useful. Continue to use coconut oil when feeding. That is, after a feed, apply a little oil on the nipple and areola, in a thin film. Before the next feed, clean the nipple and areola with a small piece of cotton soaked in water that has been boiled. So, keep bits of cotton soaked in a covered bowl of boiled water. Use a fresh piece of cotton for each breast. You are not only wiping out the oil, but also stale breast milk, perspiration, and threads from garments.

If you experience mild contractions when feeding, use your breathing for labour to deal with it. These are caused because feeding releases the oxytocin hormone which contracts the uterus and helps it to involute to its normal size. Therefore involution of the uterus is more efficient when you breastfeed.

FORERUNNER TO MILK

Towards the end of pregnancy, say in the last 3 months, women often notice a yellowish fluid escape from the breast. Even if they do not notice it, a few drops may appear and dry at the tip of the nipple, forming a crust or scab.

This is called colostrum, or foremilk. It is fed to the baby before the milk comes in Milk might take about 4 to 5 days to come in. For about 10 days it is still mixed with colostrum and looks rich and creamy. Earlier, colostrum was regarded as unclean milk, and mothers were forbidden from feeding it to the baby. This is yet another of the old wives' tales which should be ignored. Feeding colostrum to the baby is full of advantages. It definitely must be fed to the baby.

COLOSTRUM

Colostrum has a high content of fat and protein and gives the baby a full feeling. The baby remains satisfied for longer after a feed, enabling it to sleep and rest for long periods in the first days of life. This also gives the mother time to rest.

Colostrum has many antibodies. Later the baby will produce its own antibodies, but in the first few months it can't and depends on its mother for them. The colostrum, and later the breast milk, fulfil this need.

Antibodies in colostrum protect the baby from a number of bacterial and viral infections that the mother may have suffered from or has been immunized against, among these being pneumonia, whooping cough, E. coli gastroenteritis, typhoid, flu, dysentery, tetanus, etc. Although the extent of protection received by the baby may at times be complete and sometimes only partial, it is very important for the baby to get these antibodies from colostrum and mother's milk, until its body can manufacture its own antibodies, or during what is called its immunity gap.

Colostrum also has a laxative effect and helps the baby pass the first stool, which is black and sticky. The quick passage of the first stool prevents occurrence of jaundice in the baby.

It has higher cholesterol content than milk, which may be important at this stage for prompting the growth of the nervous system, and possibly later in life for helping the baby's body to process cholesterol in the body.

Colostrum further contains minerals like zinc and calcium and Vitamins A, B_6, B_{12} and E.

SECOND NIGHT SYNDROME & SKIN TO SKIN

Jan Berger, a registered nurse, has observed that 24 hours after birth, generally on the second night, babies want to be on the breast seemingly constantly. They cry if put down.

This need of the baby is not about hunger. The baby is not starving and the mother does not, not have enough milk. The baby is not manipulating the mother nor using her as a pacifier. So what is the second night about?

The second night is the baby expressing despair and confusion over being deprived of its comfortable and familiar home in the uterus.

The baby is for the first time bombarded with unfamiliar sensations. Baby feels air instead of the mother's warmth, hears sounds and voices, feels blinded by lights, may experience a few pricks. The baby is overstimulated and coping with an immature nervous system. This alters the baby's heart rate, respiratory rate and increases blood pressure. This is too much for the baby's central nervous system to handle. The baby's nervous system develops rapidly through the first year of life.

The mother, on the other hand is concentrating on health professionals like nurses and doctors, with picture shoots, friends, grandparents, siblings and other relatives. Often, the staff is telling her that the baby is too small and needs more milk, or, the baby is too large and needs more milk! They offer the bottle because 'she doesn't have anything'!

It's odd that they do not consider the medical fact that there is enough colostrum, a clear fluid, present in the breast to feed the baby for the first few days of life, and at birth, the baby's stomach capacity is just half a teaspoon.

At a time like this if we put the baby on the mother's chest, skin to skin, that is, the baby without clothes and the mother's chest without clothes, the baby and the mother, immediately calm down. One could cover them both with a sheet or the mother could be wearing a loose T-shirt.

Being skin to skin the baby feels the mother's warmth, and hears her familiar heartbeat. The mother's scent is the same as that of the amniotic fluid. This is the closest the baby can feel to being 'back home'.

In 20 minutes the baby's stress hormones are reduced by 67% and the mother's by 48%. The baby's skin temperature becomes stable.

The baby's blood glucose levels remain between 43 and 85, for a baby who has not suckled at the breast, and between 43 and 118 in a baby who has suckled at the breast.

Apart from on the second night, skin to skin contact of mother and baby should also happen at birth. Anything that separates the two should be delayed until the first breastfeed to the baby has been given.

Injections, hand prints, foot prints, photo shoots, etc. can be delayed. Any observation of the newborn by the doctor can be done while the newborn is on the mother's chest.

Giving skin to skin soothes babies, reduces crying, and reduces body movement distractions so a baby suckles more effectively. It increases the release of prolactin hormone in the mother by 33%, thus increasing the production of breastmilk. It also produces oxytocin hormone in mother and baby, causing them to bond, suppress pain, enhance sociability, improve digestion and facilitate breastfeeding; among many other advantages.

Skin to skin should be done at birth, on the second night and for the first three months of the baby's life. Premature babies and small babies especially benefit from skin to skin.

ABSENCE OF SKIN TO SKIN

When newborns are overstimulated by the environment their increased stress levels can cause them to display facial grimace, irritability, excessive alertness, frowning, arching of back, splaying of fingers, stiffening and extending limbs, turning away from eye contact, holding hands in front of face, closing eyes, inconsolability.

Newborns with high stress levels can display yawning, hiccupping, coughing, regurgitation, vomiting and touch aversion.

If the baby displays any of these signs all you need to do is skin to skin. Refrain from trying too many things. Parents tend to try one thing, then in a few minutes another thing, and in a few minutes another thing.

MATURE MILK

The colostrum gradually changes into mature milk during the first few days. There is no sudden change. The more often a baby breastfeeds, the sooner breastmilk will be produced in large amounts. It can take 3 to 5 days for the milk to come in.

In the meantime you have transitional milk, that is, milky looking colostrum. Transitional milk changes into mature milk.

Mature milk is thinner looking, whiter or bluish white. In the first year of breastfeeding, the protein present in the milk gradually falls, regardless of the mother's diet. The carbohydrates level rises, since fuel from carbohydrates is what the baby needs for development of the brain which is happening at the time.

ENGORGEMENT

A dramatic change occurs in the breasts when the milk comes in after 3 to 4 days after the delivery. The breasts become very full and hard. The change is due to the increased blood supply in the breasts and the start of full milk production. This uncomfortable stage is known as engorgement and lasts for 2 days. Some mothers who exclusively breastfeed on demand from the time of birth, do not experience engorgement.

HOW TO DEAL WITH ENGORGEMENT

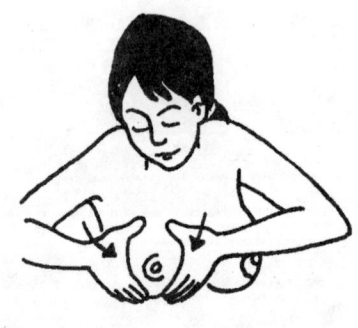

Sometimes during engorgement the baby might find it difficult to grasp the nipple and areola. In that case the mother can express some milk by pressing on the areola. This will empty the breast slightly and make it easier for the baby to grasp. However, avoid expressing milk because the more you express, the more you will produce. When engorgement happens you do not want to produce more, it will aggravate the condition.

Alternatively, a warm bath before a feed will soften the breast and help the nipple to stand out for feeding. Further, in order to make it easier for the baby to feed, you could express milk by hand or with a breastpump, just before a feed.

A cold compress will prevent engorgement by causing the blood vessels to contract. You could use wet cold towels, cooled in the refrigerator. Alternatively you could use hydrogel pads that have been chilled in the freezer, as promoted by manufacturers of breast pumps, etc. Traditionally, women have used for this purpose leaves of a cabbage, either at room temperature (in winter) or from the fridge (in summer). They wear a cold cabbage leaf inside each bra cup, and replace them as they lose their coolness. Cabbage leaves should only be used for engorgement or oversupply of milk.

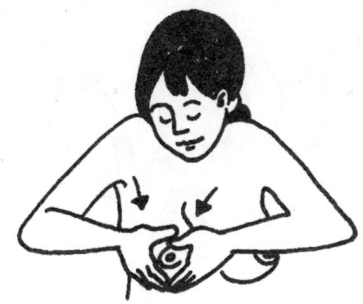

TO EXPRESS BREAST MILK

One may need to express milk when breastfeeding in a number of situations:

- To relieve engorgement so baby can grasp the nipple
- To continue feeding a sick or low birth weight baby
- To help the mother keep up her milk supply if nursing is interrupted for some reason
- To store the milk to be fed to the baby when the mother is away

To manually express milk for collection, in order to be fed later to the baby, choose a time when you are not in a hurry. Wash your hands with soap and water and dry them on a towel kept aside for this purpose. It is easier to express once the flow has begun. For instance, soon after feeding the baby from one breast, you can express from the second breast, or you could apply warmth to your breast to start the flow. During expression milk comes out slowly. The flow is greater when the baby suckles. Breast milk can also be expressed with a breast pump.

EXPRESSED MILK

Expressed milk will stay unspoilt at room temperature for 6-8 hours even in the summer. It will stay in the refrigerator for 24 hours, and in the freezer for 1 to 3 months.

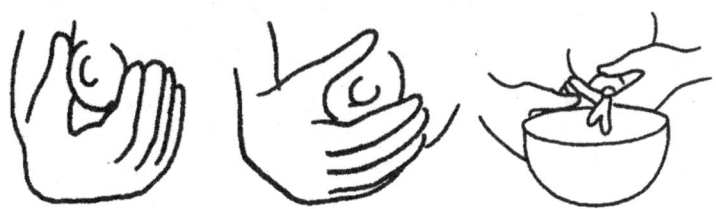

To express milk, place the thumb and fingers as flat as possible on the spot where areola and breast meet, and press. After having pressed a few times, very gently move your finger and thumb together backwards towards the chest, so that you press on the wider milk ducts behind the areola. Gradually move your thumb and finger in a circle around the areola.

BREAST PUMPS

Breast milk can also be expressed with a breast pump. There are different types of breast pumps.

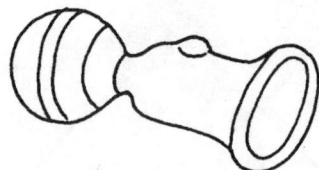

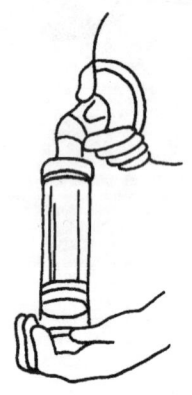

THE BULB TYPE

This has a bulb of rubber and the rest is made of a glass funnel. First the rubber bulb is pressed and the glass funnel is placed over the nipple and areola. Then the rubber bulb is released. This creates a suction and consequent release of milk. The disadvantage of this pump is that the rubber bulb cannot be boiled for sterilisation. It should only be used to remove and discard milk.

THE SYRINGE TYPE

An imported breast pump kit that works on the same principle as a syringe is available at some major chemist shops in big cities.

THE BATTERY OPERATED TYPE

These pumps are available for home use. They work well when the breast is very full.

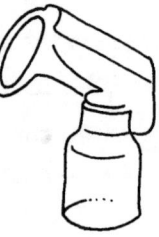

THE ELECTRIC TYPE

This is a big heavy duty pump that is generally used in hospitals.

> **STORING BREASTMILK**
>
> Whatever stainless steel glasses/bowls you are going to use for expressing, storing or feeding expressed milk can be filled with hot boiling water and left standing till you need to use it.

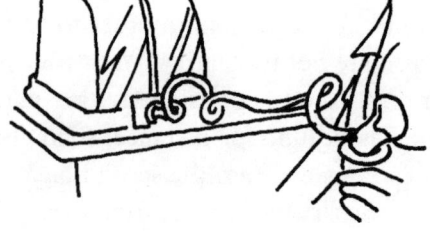

STORING BREAST MILK

While standing in the refrigerator the breast milk may separate into fat and water layers; that does not mean it has gone bad. If the milk is not really chilled, there is no harm in feeding cold milk to the baby. If expressed milk is to be fed to the baby at night, express during the morning, when milk production is greater, after you have been nicely rested. Or express at night so that it can be fed at noon the next day.

Alternatively keep collecting expressed milk by your bedside. It can be fed to the baby when required, for instance, if you sleep through a feed or are bathing when the baby wakes for a feed, or if you need to go out for a few hours.

Every 8 hours discard the remaining milk and collect in a fresh glass. If the baby's saliva has not touched the milk it can be frozen. Hence it is a good idea to store the milk in a stainless steel glass and feed from a stainless steel or silver katorie that is, a small bowl.

So if the baby does not finish the milk in the bowl, it can be discarded, since saliva has touched it. The milk in the larger glass can be used for later use.

It is best to store breast milk in a stainless steel bowl/glass. Plastic would leach chemicals into the milk, some of which are endocrine (hormone) disrupters (Vom Saal & Hughes, 2005).

In a glass made of glass, the live antibody (immunoglobin A) cells stick to the sides of the glass and the baby is deprived of them. Stainless steel containers result in a decline in cell count and cell viability. Hence the best way to feed the baby is directly from the breast. However, for storage, stainless steel is the safest option.

Before feeding, expressed breast milk should not be boiled or microwaved. Boiling will destroy its properties and a microwave heats unevenly. Just stand the bottle in hot water to warm the milk slightly and feed.

One may need to express milk when breastfeeding in a number of situations. For relief from engorgement, to continue feeding a sick or low birth weight baby, to help a mother keep up her milk supply if nursing is interrupted for some reason, or to store breast milk to feed to the baby when the mother is away.

HOW TO FEED EXPRESSED BREAST MILK

The best way of feeding expressed breast milk is directly from a glass, bowl or cup. It is best that it be made of stainless steel, and have a smooth edge. Put some expressed breast milk in the bowl. Place the baby on your lap with the head slightly raised. Place the edge of the bowl on the baby's lower lip and tilt the bowl till the level of the milk reaches the upper lip. The baby will sense its presence and lap it up with the tongue, like a puppy!

This is exactly how the baby breastfeeds. Therefore drinking from the bowl will not interfere with breastfeeding. However drinking from a bottle, spoon or a *paladi* causes confusion and the baby soon starts to prefer those methods and does not want to breastfeed thereafter. It causes confusion because these methods do not require the baby to stick its tongue out, like it needs to during breastfeeding or bowl feeding.

Babies normally take to the bowl with ease. However a baby who has already had a bottle is likely to protest against drinking from a bowl by flaying its arms. This might spill some milk, so make the baby wear a bib before trying it for the first time or ask someone to hold the baby's arms. The alternative would be to swaddle the baby or wrap it in a sheet so that its arms do not flay. Gradually the baby will become adept at it.

As the baby grows, apart from expressed breast milk, soups, juices, water, milk or any other liquid can be fed in a similar way.

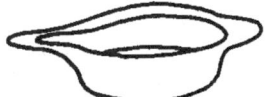

A traditional feeding cup or paladi can cause nipple confusion (see pg. 150 for "HOW TO FEED A BABY BY A CUP")

IF THE BABY'S NOSE GETS BLOCKED

If it looks like the baby's nose is getting blocked, but the baby is feeding peacefully, you don't have to do anything. It may worry you because the baby's breathing will be noisy as a result, as if the baby has a stuffy nose.

However, it is not a cause of worry; if the baby's nose is pushed back, it can still breathe. As an experiment push your nose back with your palm. You will still be able to breathe! So can the baby! Unnecessarily pressing the breast down will cause sore nipples.

Pressing the breast down will cause the nipple to project upwards. That will lead to the nipple hitting against the roof of the baby's mouth and getting sore or cracked. Thus it could result in sore or painful nipples.

Secondly, it can block the ducts on the tip of the nipple, and prevent the milk from flowing out. This could cause the baby to get agitated, since no milk will flow out. It could also cause mastitis.

Instead of pressing the breast down, place all your fingers below the breast and lift the breast. This will cause a considerable part of the bulge to tilt towards the chest and meet with the chest. It will also present the nipple at the correct angle to the baby for feeding.

If the baby's nose is blocked because of a cold you could feed the baby expressed milk from a bowl/glass. Alternatively, you can put a few drops of saline solution in the baby's nostrils to clear the block.

FEEDING TIME

The baby should be fed as and when it demands a feed. Hospital routine may encourage breastfeeds by the clock. This regulated system is based on bottle feeding, and has no bearing on breastfeeding.

The let down reflex or release of the flow of milk may take a few minutes to be established. It can be affected by embarrassment at nursing, fear of discomfort, contractions during feeding, etc. If the baby is removed too soon from the breast, the flow will be that much weaker.

In the first few days, the baby should be put to the breast as long as it likes, which could be 20 to 30 minutes at a time. The more complete the emptying of the breast, the more successful the establishment of lactation will be.

The colostrum present in the breast is heavy and the baby may not want a feed for 6 to 8 hours after having it.

Later when lactation is established, breast milk is less heavy and gaps between feeds can be 2 to 3 hours. Sometimes there could be just one hour after which the baby may want another feed!

The baby can sometimes take 40 to 60 minutes for a feed! If you are tense when feeding, the baby will sense it immediately, and may not want to leave the breast as a result. It does not mean that it is hungry; what it is doing is sucking for comfort and security.

A biochemic medicine, Kali phos 6X (to be bought from a shop selling homoeopathic medicines), can also relax the mother. She can take 4 tablets 4 times a day. On the other hand, prescription homoeopathic medicine taken from a practising homoeopath can also help you to relax.

Another time the baby may want to be breastfeeding constantly is if the baby is going through a growth spurt and needs more milk. This is Nature's way of increasing the milk supply, since the more the baby feeds the more milk gets produced. The baby may feed very frequently for a few days (the days should not exceed one week) and then settle into longer gaps again.

RELAX WHEN YOU FEED

It is important to relax when you feed. If you do not relax, it will interfere with the letting down of milk, that is, the release of milk does not take place when you are tense.

It is therefore a good idea to retire to a quiet, undisturbed corner with your baby at feeding time. You can carry with you a tall drink to savour when feeding.

Before you put the baby to the breast, calm down, sip your drink and shut your eyes for 5 to 15 minutes. You need to be undisturbed and comfortable as you do this.

If you have problems of space, you can fix a curtain in front of your bed for privacy. Or, you can use a light scarf of net or georgette to cover yourself and your baby.

If you have a room to yourself, restrict the entry of guests when feeding. Sometimes free entry of staff or extended family can hamper the release of milk.

Like all things intimate, breastfeeding requires privacy and forgetting the clock. One should feed on demand, that is, let the baby decide when it needs a feed; whether it wants a short gap or a long gap between feeds. This is called 'baby-led feeding'.

NIGHT FEED

Newborn babies need to be fed frequently, because of their body weight and their fast rate of growth. Until the baby weighs around 10 pounds it will need to wake up at night for a feed. Once the baby weighs 10 pounds it can sleep for about 5 hours without waking up with hunger.

Try and give the baby the last feed when you yourself go to bed at night. When the baby wakes up at night, you can feed the baby in bed, and let him drop off to sleep with you. Keep a nappy change, and a torch close at hand. Instead of a torch, you can keep a zero watt bulb switched on all night.

Do not delay the feed until the baby cries. If the baby is allowed to cry when he is hungry, it will fray your nerves; besides, when put to the breast, the baby will feed only for a short while and fall asleep from exhaustion; only to wake up with hunger after an hour or so.

So when your baby wakes up for a feed at night, pick him up, or have your husband pass him to you. Your husband can help you in this way at least 3 times a week. Keep the room darkened. Do not play or otherwise distract the baby. Sing a lullaby, which should be sung only at bedtime. Let the baby learn to associate minimum activity with night-time.

At least 3 times a week go to bed early if your baby regularly wakes up at night. Keep water by your bedside in case you get thirsty. Also keep some food in case you get hungry. If you find it difficult to go back to sleep, try to relax by totally letting go your body, closing your eyes and letting your thoughts run as they will. Watch your thoughts as though you are watching a movie, that is, without judgement.

Make sure you are comfortable, your clothes are comfortable, the temperature in your room is comfortable, the position you are in is comfortable.

If you are very tired, you can express breast milk which can be fed to the baby by your husband through a bowl. This will enable you to sleep through one feed and get 4 to 5 hours of undisturbed sleep. It is recommended that this is made routine since a mother who is well rested can cope better with the demands of motherhood. The baby will also relax if he senses the mother's relaxed mood.

FOREMILK AND HIND MILK

The early part of a feed is made up of foremilk which is low in fat, while the latter part is the hind milk which has 4 to 5 times the amount of fat and 1½ times as much protein. Hence the foremilk is thin, whereas hind milk is thicker.

Many mothers who feed their babies from both breasts at one feed, think they are not producing enough milk. Their baby gets only the thin, low-calorie foremilk, and the mother stops feeding before the high-fat hindmilk is consumed by the baby. As a result, the baby actually loses weight or fails to gain weight and is therefore started on supplements by the anxious parents. It is therefore important to feed from one breast mostly at one feed. The fat-rich milk also gives more satisfaction to the baby so that he demands the next feed after bigger gaps.

HOW TO TELL IF THE BABY IS HUNGRY

Some mothers wait for the baby to cry for a feed. They consider it to be a signal that the baby is hungry.

However, when the baby cries, it means that the baby is desperate for a feed and has reached the end of its patience. At such times the baby may then be too upset and exhausted to feed properly. He may fall asleep after having just a little bit of milk to satisfy hunger pangs. Not having had a full feed, he will wake up again fairly quickly for another feed. Therefore do not wait for the baby to cry, look for signs that the baby is ready to feed.

Look for feeding cues or signs that a baby is hungry or else you will have a hungry and angry baby on your hands. A crying baby will move a lot, turn red in colour and stretch the limbs or arch the back. Sucking helps to clam a crying baby before feeding. After washing your hands, allow the baby to suck your little finger, fleshy side up. This will calm the baby and make it ready for a feed.

These are some of the signs that mean that the baby is ready for a feed:

1. The baby may make small noises
2. The Baby may be wakeful and restless
3. The Baby may make hand to mouth movements
4. The Baby may make sucking movements
5. The Baby may suck its fingers
6. The baby may turn to a side, with the mouth open. This is called the 'rooting reflex', can also be called mouthing
7. Tongue protrusion
8. Lip smacking

WILL MY MILK BE ENOUGH?

Since we cannot measure the number of ounces of milk a breastfed baby gets, many mothers wonder whether it is enough. Remember, it is Nature's food for the baby, the same Nature that nourished the baby inside the womb and made it form into a little human being. Your milk is the best suited to your baby's needs, much as cow's milk is best suited to a calf's needs.

To check if the baby is getting adequate nourishment, the doctor will weigh the baby when you go for a check-up. If your doctor says the baby is putting on weight normally, it is obvious that your milk is sufficient.

It is also important to know that all babies lose weight in the first 7 to 10 days of life. They take the same number of days to regain their birth weight. Then their weight gain begins.

For the first 2 days approximately, a full-term baby may sleep a lot and not want many feeds, if it is warm and well. After a suckle at the breast in these initial days the baby can sleep for about 8 hours without wanting a feed!

From the third to seventh day, the baby may want to feed more frequently in order to establish the milk supply.

Once the milk supply is established babies feed less frequently, but their habits can vary. Any baby may want to feed more on some days and less on other days.

If the baby does not suckle at the breast and neither does the mother express milk, milk secretion will stop. There is a substance which can reduce or inhibit milk production. If a lot of milk is left in the breast, the inhibitor stops the cells from secreting milk anymore. So do not, not feed in the hope of collecting more milk for the next feed.

LESS MILK

If you feel you are producing less milk, all you have to do is feed more often. Each time you feed, the body releases prolactin hormones, which further stimulate the production of milk.

If you skip a feed in the hope of storing more milk for the next feed, it will not work, for the less you feed, the more your milk supply will dwindle.

> **HOW TO TELL IF BABY IS GETTING ENOUGH MILK**
>
> After one week of life if a baby has 6 wet diapers and soft, abundant stool in 24 hours, it is getting enough input, or milk. Besides, less volume of breast milk is needed as compared to other milk because all of breast milk gets absorbed, unlike formula milk.

The amount consumed at a feed can be determined by weighing the baby before and after a feed without a change of clothes.

It has been noted that 'less milk' is often a complaint at two to two and a half months. Possibly because by then overfilling and leaking of breast milk does not happen, and the breasts become smaller. However if the baby's weight gain is adequate, it is not a cause for worry.

It you feel the milk is not enough, feed more often and persist. If you get panicky and mix breast with bottle, the battle is lost. For the baby soon starts preferring the bottle to the breast. Bottle feeding requires less effort on the baby's part. Mothers feel reassured with the bottle since they can measure the amount of milk the baby has had.

There are certain foods called 'galactogogues' that are believed to increase milk production. It is said that eating *jeera* or cumin seeds, *methi* or fenugreek seeds increases the production of milk.

Frequent breastfeeds and drinking lots of water also helps.

You should check with your doctor about any medicine you take, just to make sure it will not affect the milk supply.

BURPING THE BABY

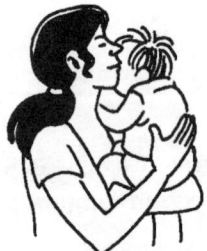

Babies should be made to burp once or twice during a feed. The baby can burp once while being fed and later at the end of a feed. With the burp the baby could bring up some milk or curd.

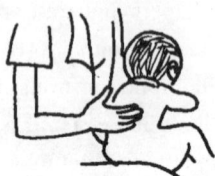

Burping brings up any wind that has been swallowed during feeding or crying prior to feeding, so that it does not cause any discomfort to the baby. Babies vary a great deal in the amount of air they swallow, so some may burp immediately, while others take longer to burp. Bottle-fed babies swallow more air than breastfed babies. So do breastfed babies who gulp milk fast or cry while feeding. If not burped, the baby can become uncomfortable and restless. However, if the baby does not burp when held upright in order to be made to burp, and seems otherwise happy and satisfied, do not become particular about burping. Let it pass. Probably she has not swallowed much air.

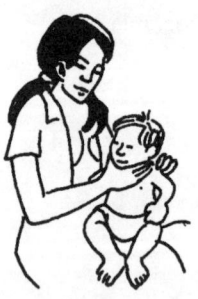

If the baby falls asleep while having a feed, do not wake her up for burping. Put her on its side. This position will cause the air to come up automatically. The milk she brings up with a burp will run out of the mouth and not bother her.

HOW TO POSITION THE BABY

Correct positioning of the baby for breastfeeding can actually determine the success or failure of breastfeeding!

A correctly positioned baby will feed effortlessly without causing pain to the mother. Besides, the mother will not suffer from back and shoulder pain as a result of breastfeeding.

There are some basic guidelines for how the mother needs to position herself and the baby for successful breastfeeding.

HICCUPS

Sometimes babies start hiccuping after a feed. It is nothing to worry about, although some parents get anxious when they hear the baby's rather loud hiccups. It is normal and will pass.

Firstly the mother's back should be straight and supported either by the back of a chair, a wall or the headboard of the bed.

She should hold the baby to her breast sideways, so that the baby's tummy is opposite her body, and the baby's nose is opposite her nipple. That is, the baby needs to be held fairly low.

Then she should touch the baby's lips with her nipple. Wait for the baby to open her mouth wide, with the tongue protruding; then quickly pull the baby close so that the baby gets a big mouthful of breast in her wide open mouth.

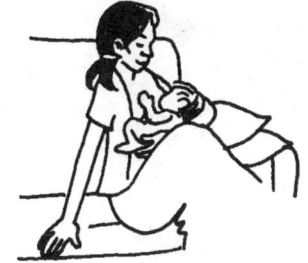

This ensures that the baby's gums press on the areola, the dark area behind the nipple and not on the nipple. By doing so the baby presses on the area where the sinuses of milk are, as a result of which the milk reaches the baby's mouth through the nipple, and goes straight down the baby's throat.

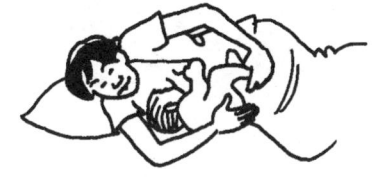

This process is interfered with if the mother presses the top part of her breast to prevent the baby's nose from getting blocked by her breast.

If the mother does so, the nipple, instead of going towards the baby's throat, gets directed to the roof of the baby's mouth. On hitting the roof of the baby's mouth the nipple could get sore and painful. Or, the milk fails to be released from the tip of the nipple as the roof of the baby's mouth blocks it! This can cause the baby to leave the breast and cry in frustration.

So the mother must never press her breast down even if the baby's nose looks like it is getting blocked, and the baby's breathing is noisy.

It will help if the mother can get support for her elbows as she feeds. For instance, if she can support her elbows on an armrest of a chair.

Alternatively, she can be sitting on the bed, against the headboard, with pillows to support the baby and her elbows.

Basically, the mother should take a back-rest and sit with her back straight. It may not be possible for her to sit straight after the birth of the baby, because her pelvic floor may be uncomfortable. In that case she can sit between two pillows.

Alternatively, when the mother is tired at night, she can lie down on her side and feed the baby. It is important for the mother to be relaxed in whichever position she adopts.

When the mother is feeding, she should take care to see that the breast falls towards the baby. If the breast is falling away from the baby, it will require the baby to tug at the nipple and may cause soreness or cracks in the nipples.

POSITION AFTER CAESAREAN BIRTH

If the baby has been delivered under general anesthesia, the mother is likely to be unconscious initially. As soon as the mother responds to commands (that is, if she is told to move to her right or left, she responds), breastfeeding can be started, as described below.

After epidural anesthesia the mother can start breastfeeding within 30 minutes of birth. The sooner she does so, the better.

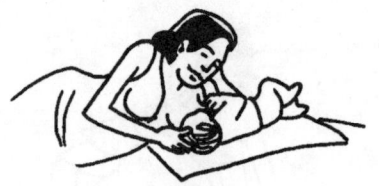
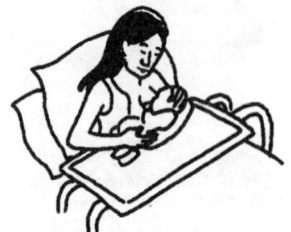
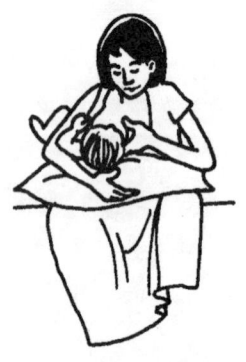
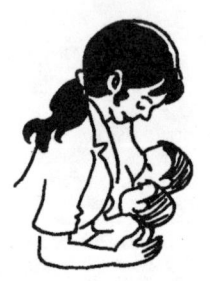
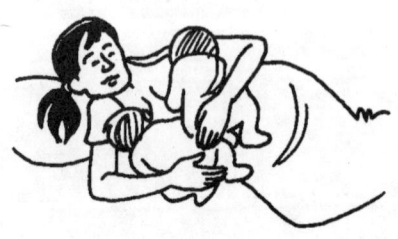

After epidural anesthesia, the mother is asked to lie on her back for 24 hours after the birth of the baby.

As soon as possible after birth by Caesarean section, the baby can be placed on top of the mother for feeding.

As the mother lies on her back, the baby can be placed over her, with the baby's head towards her right or left breast, and the baby's feet towards her right or left shoulder.

Or, the baby can be placed at her right breast with feet tapering towards her left breast, across her body.

Thirdly, the baby could be placed on the side, with feet on the bed and head at the breast.

Do not place the baby at the breast with feet towards the mother's legs. That can cause the baby's feet to touch the Caesarean scar and cause discomfort to the mother.

When the mother can sit, the baby can be placed on one side of the mother, under her armpit. The baby's tummy should turn towards the mother's waist and the baby's feet should taper towards the mother's back.

When her stitches have healed she can also lie down and feed, or hold the baby in front and feed.

TWINS

Twins can be fed one at a time, or together. When two babies suck at the breasts, the breasts produce enough milk to feed both.

You can feed twins 3 hourly rather than feeding them on demand. In the beginning, you can feed each baby separately, so that you can get to know them individually. You can feed them one after the other. Start with whoever wakes up first and then wake the other baby. Many twin babies develop a preference for their own breast. One baby might be an eager sucker while the other may be lazy.

HOW TO POSITION TWINS

Place a pillow on your lap below the breast. Place the baby's head at the breast, and let the baby's body taper to the side of your body, the feet falling to the side of your waist, under your arm. Place the other baby on the other breast in a similar fashion.

Or else, you can place a baby in the usual way, that is, head at one breast, and the body tapering towards the other breast, and the second baby with the body tapering towards the side of your body.

BONDING

The more skin-to-skin contact your baby enjoys with your body when feeding, the more strong a bond will develop between you and the baby. You should hold the baby against your bare skin when feeding.

If you haven't felt very motherly at birth, you are going to feel a gush of maternal affection as your baby gazes intently straight into your eyes when feeding. This is specially important if you have had a Caesarean birth.

You can also hold an adopted baby against your skin as you bottle-feed it. Or you can hold a surrogate baby likewise.

Babies also tend to grasp your finger, or, when older, scratch or stroke your breast when feeding. As they feel relaxed and satisfied at the breast, they begin to play around with their mother's necklace or chain.

CONTRACEPTIVE EFFECTS OF BREASTFEEDING

Breastfeeding is more likely to have a contraceptive effect if the mother is breastfeeding exclusively through the day and night. That is, she is not giving the baby any other milk or water.

When the mother breastfeeds in this way, she is also likely not to have a menstrual period.

Both of the above are likely to be the case within the first 6 months of the child's life. Therefore, if a mother is exclusively breastfeeding a baby less than 6 months of age, and not having a period, her chances of becoming pregnant are as low as 2%. Each time she feeds the baby she releases prolactin, a hormone that suppresses ovulation.

BREAST OR BOTTLE

The advantages of breastfeeding undoubtedly far outweigh bottle-feeding. Sometimes the bottle may be resorted to for some reason. There is no need to feel guilty if that is the case. The aim of both is a well-nourished, happy and active baby.

At times bottle-feeding may be resorted to if the mother is working. In that case the baby can still take one or two breastfeeds, early morning and late at night.

If the baby does not gain adequate weight bottle-feeding is often resorted to. However, the mother should also be reminded that the hind milk or the last part of the breast milk is rich in fat. If the initial watery milk is 20% fat, the hind milk is 50% fat. Babies who are fed the hind milk sleep well and grow healthy. The fat content increases gradually towards the end of the feed. If the mother feeds from one breast at one feed for 20 to 30 minutes, constantly, the baby is likely to get the fat rich-hind milk.

At times recurrent cracking of nipples, mastitis, or surgery for the mother might lead to a switch.

An exhausted mother, unable to cope with demand feeding and other household chores, may get so tired and anxious that it might interfere with her lactation. It is therefore advisable to arrange for extra help at this time.

A woman may have in-laws, friends, or a husband who are not very enthusiastic about breastfeeding. On the other hand, some women may give up breastfeeding due to wrong advice or hearsay; for example, some women believe breastfeeding ruins their figures. There is no credibility in this, as it

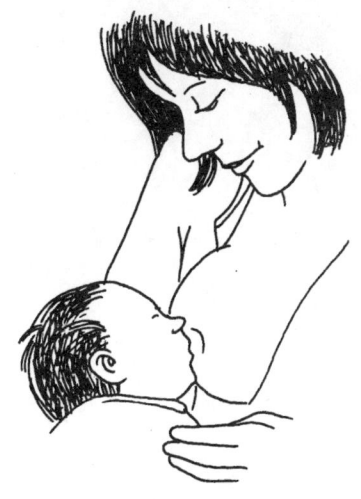

CALORIE CONTENT OF BREAST MILK

Foremilk 1.5 cal/ounce
Hind milk 25-30 cal/ounce

Source: Dr Richard Applebaum, Nursing your Baby

has been seen from medical experience that many women breastfeed several babies with no effects on their figure. Others end up with even better figures. Very few women give up breastfeeding for the reasons listed above. Basically, if a woman decides to breastfeed, she normally succeeds. Most mothers give up because they feel they have fed long enough or as long as they had planned.

A breastfed baby is not prone to allergies. There are less chances of diarrhoea, eczema, coughs, colds, and asthma in breastfed babies.

Some women fear feeding will make them less sexy. This is not true, since sex, childbirth and breastfeeding are linked with the same hormone. Many women feel more sexy when feeding.

It is easier to breastfeed if you are travelling. No hassles of sterilizing bottles and running around to find a place to make feeds. All you need is yourself and maybe a shawl or scarf to cover yourself.

HOW LONG SHOULD ONE FEED LAST?

A baby takes approximately 20 minutes of constant sucking to empty a breast. However if the baby periodically falls asleep when feeding, the feed can last longer. Sometimes mothers say the baby feeds for as long as 45 to 60 minutes. That is why it is important to not pay too much attention to the time. Simply feed till the baby is satisfied and has no desire to feed any more.

If the mother is relaxed, when she breastfeeds, the baby is likely to have a good feed and release the breast sooner.

The following factors will help a mother to breastfeed:

- The mother has privacy, she should not be watched when breastfeeding.
- The mother is not stressed with constant knocks on the door or visitors.
- The mother has nutritious food and liquids.
- The mother is not constantly asked about her success at breastfeeding.
- The mother is not distracted by the phone or computer.
- The mother has the baby next to her, in her bed, or in the cot.
- There are not too many people in the room, e.g. grandmother, aunt, nurse, maid, cousin, etc., each with their differing thoughts or instructions.
- The mother has minimum household responsibility.
- The mother has the will to breastfeed.
- The mother has previous information on how to breastfeed and position the baby.
- The mother and family do not panic in the first 3 to 4 days when there is only colostrum in the breast.
- The mother and family do not panic when engorgement happens.

HOW LONG TO BREASTFEED?

Exclusive breastfeeding is recommended for 6 months. After 6 months complementary feeding of weaning foods can be started along with breastfeeding. Ideally a baby should be breastfed for 2 years; or, for a minimum of 6 months.

Some mothers feed for 1 year or 8 months. The reason why breastfeeding is recommended for 2 years is that it gives the baby greater immunity to fight infection during the teething phase. At that time the baby will be eating other food, and breastfeeding may be just once or twice a day. Also, if the mother is an airhostess or a doctor, her duty hours could be 24 hours or longer, in that case the bottle will have to be resorted to.

BREASTFEEDING AND THE WORKING WOMAN

BREAST TO BOTTLE

If you know you have to go back to work soon, e.g. in three months, combine breastfeeding and bottle-feeding a few weeks before you rejoin work. Start with one bottle of expressed milk in the morning around 10 a.m. i.e. the time you are likely to be away. Start introducing a routine, in which you gradually cut out breastfeeds and introduce bottle-feeds instead during your working hours. You could continue to breastfeed before and after working hours.

After 6 months you can also introduce mashed bananas (slightly overripe) and bland preparations of khichadi/kheer/halwa/upma/any dal without tarka, with a little ghee/mashed potato.

If your work is going to require you to be away for a few days on and off, switch to the bottle totally by the 3rd month.

BOTTLE TO BREASTFEED

If you want to increase the number of breastfeeds and reduce the number of bottle-feeds, breastfeeding more often will cause the release of prolactin hormone and an increase in breast milk production.

Each time you are to give a bottle-feed, first put the baby to the breast, and then give the other milk from a glass. Gradually, in the next few days your own milk supply will build up and you will not need the other milk at all.

Many women ask what they can eat or drink to increase breast milk supply! Taking plenty of fluids will help increase milk supply, for example, water, nimbupani, soup, coconut water.

Traditionally, foods that are meant to increase breast milk supply are porridge/dalia, red egyptian lentil/lal masoor dal, cumin/jeera seeds, ginger/adrak and in the West a glass of beer, which is very effective.

CASE AGAINST THE BOTTLE

Bottle-feeding should be resorted to only when absolutely necessary. Its potential hazards must be borne in mind. If the milk is not made properly, it can mean a sick baby. Besides, bottle-feeding requires a lot of hard work. One has to sterilize the feeding bottles, nipples, etc. This is very important.

QUICKIES

In order to reduce preparation time before a feed, or to be able to carry a quickie food while travelling, the following ready mix powder can be kept handy. Take some rice grains and lightly roast them on the tawa or in a cooking vessel over the fire. When roasted cool them and dry-grind them in a mixie, so that you get ready cooked rice powder. Bottle it. When required you can add water, milk, watery dal/or any other liquid to it and feed the baby. You could do the same with other grains like ragi, bajra, jowar, wheat, etc.

Along with these cereals, you can also roast pulses or dals and nuts; and dry-grind them also and mix with the cereals.

If sterilizing is not done properly, it can cause diarrhoea and dehydration in the baby.

Once you start with bottle-feeding, the baby may begin to prefer it and start rejecting the breast. The baby may even want breast milk only from the bottle!

When the baby drinks directly from the breast, it signals to the mother's body the current needs of the baby. So if the baby is dehydrated or feverish the constituents of the mother's milk will change to cater to those requirements. For instance, more antibodies to fight the fever will be added to the milk. Or, if the baby is dehydrated, more water will be added to the milk.

The contraceptive effect of breastfeeding will also be less without exclusive breastfeeding.

If you give a bottle-feed at night, you will have to be fully alert and awake to make a bottle-feed and bring it to the right temperature. It is easier to simply put the baby to the breast. Each bottle-feed has to be made manually.

THE BOTTLE AND NIPPLE CONFUSION

Feeding the baby from the bottle causes nipple confusion, and should be avoided. At the breast the baby needs to work hard with its jaw to feed. The bottle, on the other hand, drips milk regardless of the baby's jaw effort. The baby gets used to this easy flow from the bottle's nipple and dislikes working hard at the breast's nipple.

The disadvantage of the constant flow of the bottle's nipple is that the baby needs to suck and swallow quickly. This results in a respiratory load on the child and is not recommended at all for small babies or premature babies. It would be similar to your being asked to finish a bottle of water or cola without a break. It would leave you gasping for breath. Small or premature babies can be tube-fed, then cup/glass-fed (cup-feeding can start from 29 weeks or 7 months and one week gestation) and finally breastfed.

In this sequence of feeding they will breastfeed with ease. It avoids nipple confusion.

Further, the baby gets used to overfeeding when drinking from the bottle. This can sow the seeds of overeating and obesity.

MILK POWDER

Making a powdered-milk feed should be done exactly according to the instructions on the tin. Some people put extra milk powder in the feed, since they feel the milk looks very thin. This could be dangerous. It could lead to a concentration of minerals in the baby's bloodstream, which can lead to dehydration and illness.

On the other hand, some people might put less milk powder as compared to the instructions on the tin, thus running the risk of providing inadequate nourishment to the baby.

You must discuss with your doctor which is the best milk to give the baby. If you are going to be travelling a lot, it is best to give powdered milk, so that there are less frequent changes, since you can carry the milk powder with you wherever you go. Besides, it is sterilized and does not become easily infected. The brand you use should not be changed; it is best to stick to one brand.

When making a feed, a little extra milk can be prepared in case the baby wants to have a little extra.

If it is not consumed, the extra milk should be thrown away after a feed.

Milk can be made in a large jug and kept covered in the refrigerator for not more than 24 hours. Little quantities of it can be transferred to sterilized bottles when needed. Or, milk can be poured into sterilized bottles and kept in the refrigerator. When needed, it can be removed and warmed by using a bottle warmer or by standing the bottle in mug of hot water before use. It is a good rule to follow, rather than letting someone else make the milk.

COW'S MILK

Cow's milk has more protein than mother's milk. This unnaturally large intake of protein results in a large load of nitrogen for the infant's kidneys. Cow's milk should therefore be given diluted with one part water to three parts of cow's milk. The water dilutes the protein and minerals like sodium and nitrogen.

A little sugar should be added to the milk, since mother's milk has more carbohydrate than cow's milk.

HOW TO STERILIZE BOTTLES

You must keep aside a large vessel in the kitchen for boiling bottles in. You can buy one with a lid, since a covered vessel uses up less fuel. You will also need a bottle brush, which you must make sure is kept clean. Some people use electric steam sterilizers.

Unscrew the covers of the bottles. Separate nipples. In order to get the slime off the nipples, rinse them in water, then apply salt inside and outside them and put them in the sun on a plate.

Wash the bottles, rims and covers of the bottles.

Use a liquid dishwashing soap or a soapy solution of a clothes washing detergent. Scrub them well on the inside with a bottle cleaning brush, to remove the slime that milk tends to leave behind. If left behind, the slime forms a breeding ground for germs. You could fill used bottles with water after use so that milk does not dry in them and they are easier to clean. When the bottles are nicely scrubbed clean, fill them with water before you immerse them in the vessel of water, so that you have a minimum number of air bubbles in the bottles and they remain nicely submerged. Alternatively place them in the electric sterilizer.

When all parts of the bottle are scrubbed and immersed in water, put the vessel on the flame, with the lid on. When the water boils, it will send up steam and bubbles of air, and make a gurgling sound. It is important that this stage

HOW TO STERILISE BOTTLES

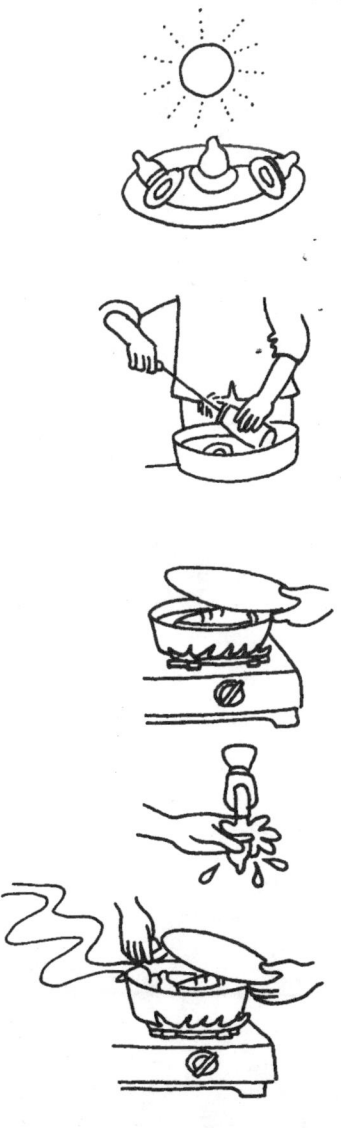

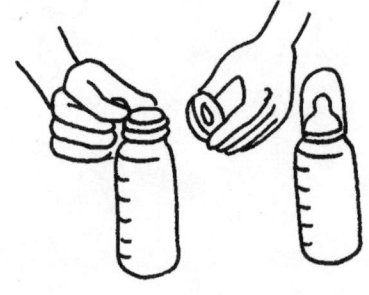

is reached, for only when the water boils actively do the germs get killed.

When the water is boiling, bring the nipples inside and wash them thoroughly in running water, to remove every trace of salt. It should not be left behind in the nipple, since the baby should not get an unnecessary extra daily dosage of salt. Then remove the lid of the vessel, put the nipples in the vessel and turn off the flame after a couple of minutes.

When the water is cool enough to handle, wash your hands with soap and remove the feeding equipment. Fix the nipples on the rims, and put the covers on the bottles and keep aside for use during the day.

If you have to go out to work, you can make the milk and pour it into individual covered or sealed bottles and leave behind in the refrigerator, so that it can be fed while you are away.

HOW TO BOTTLE-FEED

The baby, while being bottle-fed, should be held close as in breastfeeding. Do not place the baby on the bed and feed it like a doll. Bottle-feeding should not only provide nourishment, but also warmth and security to the child. You can also hold the baby next to your naked skin. This is specially important if the baby has been separated from you earlier on, on account of illness, premature birth or any other reason. The mutual feedback you and your baby get from each other at this time will build a new relationship and bond between you both.

Before giving the bottle, check the temperature of the milk by letting a few drops of milk fall on the back of your hand from the bottle. If the milk feels pleasantly warm, it is the right temperature. If it feels hot, cool it by waiting a little or placing the bottle in cold water. If the milk is made and kept in the refrigerator in sterilized bottles, there is no harm in giving the baby cold milk. If it is winter and the milk from the fridge is too cold, it can be stood in a mug of hot water before being fed to the baby.

If during a feed you have to keep the bottle aside for a little while, cover it with a special cap that comes with feeding bottles. Do not let the nipple be exposed to flies and do not cover it with your hanky or towel. Avoid touching the nipple with the fingers.

When feeding, hold the baby upright, that is, head higher than the rest of the body. Hold the bottle firmly at a slant, and make sure the nipple reaches way back in the baby's mouth. The nipple should always be full of milk, or else the baby will take in too much air and have a lot of wind. If the teat flattens and the milk stops going through, pull the bottle gently backwards to release the vacuum.

Check if the nipple's hole is large enough. When the bottle is inverted, it should allow several drops to flow in one second. If you find the flow is very slow, enlarge the hole with a red-hot needle. Hold the tip of the needle in a flame, and when it becomes red-hot in colour with the heat, pierce the tip of the nipple with it.

Let the baby have a pause during a feed, now and then. Burp the baby.

PROBLEMS DURING BREASTFEEDING

WHEN THE BABY CHOKES

If a mother has too much milk that flows too fast, the baby might choke on it. In case this happens, the mother should express a little milk before feeding the baby.

Sometimes the baby may choke if the mother's nipples are too big and long. The baby may turn its head away from the breast and cry, moving its arms and legs. In this case, the mother should hold the baby a little away from the breast.

SORE NIPPLES

When you want to stop feeding, if you pull and drag the baby off the breast, it might give you sore nipples. Instead, you must break the baby's suction by putting the tip of your finger in the corner of the mouth between the gums, and then take it off the breast.

Or, pull the chin downwards.

If you press your breast down with the finger, by forming a big dent on the breast, in order to prevent the baby's nose from getting blocked, the act of pressing the breast down will cause the nipple to project upwards and hit the roof of the baby's mouth when it feeds. This hitting of the nipple on the hard palate will cause it to get sore. Besides, it will block the release of milk from the front tip of the nipple.

Soreness sometimes occurs if the nipples are frequently washed with soap and water. Water is sufficient to wash them with. Pressure applied at the same point constantly can also lead to soreness. It therefore helps to change positions during a feed and to adopt different positions for different feeds, so that pressure is applied to different points on the breast.

HOW TO HEAL SORE NIPPLES

Soggy nipples, that is, nipples that remain wet for long periods, are prone to soreness. It therefore helps to expose your nipples to air and sunlight as much as possible, until the soreness heals. You can wear a loose garment without a bra.

Avoid using creams on cracked nipples. The sore area needs to breathe in order to heal. Cream or oil will prevent the 'breathing' of the wound.

Calendula Q, as mentioned in the box on this page, can be used to provide healing. It can be wiped off with cotton and previously boiled water before a feed. After the crack has healed you can resume using oil on the nipple after a feed and wipe with wet cotton before a feed.

It is also very helpful to express some milk after a feed and rub it on the sore nipple where it should be left to dry. This quickens healing considerably. Avoid the use of waterproof-backed bra pads. Do not remove any crust appearing on the nipple. It is part of the healing process. Always offer the less sore side

HOME REMEDY

You could dab the sore area with cotton soaked in water to which a few drops of calendula Q, a homoeopathic medicine has been added, and leave it to dry.

first. That will establish the flow on the sore side before the baby takes it, thus making it less painful. You can use breathing for labour to be able to handle the pain. An aspirin or a mild alcoholic drink (beer or wine) taken shortly before a feed will help reduce the pain. It can be taken if the pain begins to interfere with the release or flow of milk.

Try using a cold compress on your nipples before feeding. Apply an ice cube wrapped in a towel or a hanky, for about 5 to 10 minutes.

Sometimes, a sore nipple may bleed. There is no harm if the baby swallows tiny amounts of blood with the milk. This can be quite frightening, especially when the baby burps after a feed, and along with the curdled milk brings up a little blood. However, this is harmless to the baby.

THRUSH/CANDIDA INFECTION

(PAIN SHOOTS INTO BREAST WHEN FEEDING)

Candida infection can happen after the use of antibiotics to treat mastitis or other infection.

In the baby this infection manifests as white patches on the baby's tongue or inside the baby's mouth. These white patches cannot be wiped off.

In the mother it may show up as a shiny red area of the nipple and areola. Sometimes the nipple/areola may lose some pigmentation i.e. look lighter in colour. The skin may also feel sore and itchy, or become flaky. In some mothers the nipples continue to look normal.

Mothers with candida can have a burning, stinging sensation that continues after a feed.

Occasionally, mothers say that when they breastfeed a pain shoots deep into the breast. The pain is present even though the baby is well latched at the breast. In agony, the mother may want to immediately take the baby off the breast. The pain feels like needles are being driven into the breast.

In case candida is suspected, one must immediately stop the use of pacifiers, teats and nipple shields. If used, they should be boiled for 20 minutes daily and replaced weekly.

Mother and baby both need to be treated together. They can be treated with gentian violet or nystatin.

Gentian violet is a purple liquid that can make it look very messy, but it is an excellent remedy.

TREATING THRUSH/CANDIDA

BABY	MOTHER
USE	USE
0.25% **Gentian violet paint**	0.5% **Gentian violet paint**
Apply in baby's mouth	Apply on mother's nipple
FREQUENCY	FREQUENCY
Daily or on alternate days	Daily
DURATION	DURATION
For 5 days or 3 days after lesions have healed	5 days

OR

BABY	MOTHER
USE **Nystatin suspension** 100,000 IU/G Apply 1 ml by dropper to child's mouth	USE **Nystatin cream** 100,000 IU/G Apply to mother's nipple
FREQUENCY 4 times daily after breastfeed	FREQUENCY 4 times daily after breastfeed
DURATION For 7 days or till mother is being treated	DURATION Continue to apply for 7 days after lesions have healed

Source: Breastfeeding Promotion Network of India (BPNI)

BLOCKED DUCTS

The signs of a blocked duct are a painful reddish area on the breast or areola. It feels sore and can be accompanied by a hot and shivery feeling, chills, bodyache and a feeling of being unwell. Sometimes there may be fever of 101° F or higher.

Let us understand why this happens. There are a number of ducts in the breasts. They carry milk produced in the milk-producing cells in the breast, towards the nipple and areola (dark-skinned area behind the nipples) to make milk available to the baby when it sucks.

If any of these ducts get blocked and milk is not able to flow through them, it results in blocked ducts. If a blocked duct is unattended, it can cause mastitis in the mother. However, dealing with a blocked duct as mentioned below prevents mastitis.

Blocked ducts may be caused by

- Incomplete emptying of the breast
- Physical pressure on the breast, e.g. from constantly having the same position when breastfeeding, a tight bra, an underwire bra, from a sleeping position, holding the baby too tightly against the breast, or your fingers may press a duct and block it if you are pressing the breast during a feed.
- Sometimes very large breasts may hang in a way that the ducts on the lower part may not flow freely. In this case lifting the breast could help.

HOW TO DEAL WITH A BLOCKED DUCT

Gentle but firm massage of the swelling towards the nipple during a feed and after, if the block is still there, will help.

Do not stop breastfeeding. Offer the non-affected side first, in order to establish the flow of milk. As soon as the flow is established, offer the affected breast to ensure vigorous sucking and drainage of the blocked duct.

Lean forward over the baby as you feed, so that gravity also aids the process. Give the baby extra feeds from the affected breast. Express the remaining milk after a feed.

Mothers should also make sure the bra is not tight, especially if the bra has a band across the top of the breast when the flap is open. Avoid underwire bras, or anything that presses the breast.

Get plenty of rest. Actually go to bed for a day. Exercise the arms, shoulders, and upper half of the body; it may help disperse the swelling caused by the blocked duct.

After practising the above, a mother should feel better in 24 hours. If she does not, she should seek medical help.

MASTITIS (INFLAMMATION OF THE BREAST)

There are two kinds of mastitis associated with lactation: Superficial Mastitis and Acute Intra-mammary Mastitis.

Superficial mastitis appears like a boil at the margin of the areola. The boil enlarges, becomes a swelling and may eventually form an abscess.

It helps if the breast is frequently emptied either through breastfeeding, which can be continued, or through expression of breastmilk.

Early start of antibiotics can cure the condition completely. However, once a lump forms, even as small as 2 mm, it mostly needs to be surgically cleaned out. If there is no improvement after 4 days of antibiotics it is best to go for surgical drainage.

Acute intra-mammary Mastitis generally happens after 5 days of birth, within the first few weeks. Gland tissue inside the breast gets inflamed. It is most likely to occur in breasts that are overproducing and congested. Sometimes it occurs after abrupt weaning.

The signs: the mother notices that one part of her breast has become painful, tender and hard. The overlying skin is red. She may have transient fever.

If not treated with frequent feeding or emptying of the breast and antibiotics and analgesics the symptoms worsen, the fever returns and an abscess develops—making the mother much more ill.

It is important to understand that the infection is due to congestion and stagnation in the breast, therefore milk must be removed. Breastfeeding the baby or expressing milk alone will help the condition, as well as enable breastfeeding to continue after recovery.

PREVENTION OF MASTITIS

To avoid mastitis the lactating mother should be alert to any change in her breasts in the form of red patches or unusual hardness, which is different from the overall hardness of a breast full of milk.

To avoid blocked ducts and engorgement, keep the breasts well-drained. This can be done by feeding the baby regularly and frequently, and by expressing any surplus milk that makes the breast uncomfortable. It can be done with the hands or with the aid of a breast pump.

Applebaum (1970) recommends that the baby should suck twice as often on the affected breast. He claims that if you can do this in addition to giving antibacterial and analgesics, weaning is never necessary and abscess formation rare.

Sometimes the mother becoming cold could lead to blocked ducts, because it causes circulatory changes in the breasts or because the change of temperature in the mammary gland, changes its bacterial environment. A breastfeeding mother should therefore remain warm and comfortable.

BREAST ABSCESS

Failure to treat mastitis, or unnecessary weaning after mastitis may lead to a breast abscess. The lump of a breast abscess can be red/hard/painful. When examined, the swelling of the abscess appears to be full of fluid.

It requires treatment by antibiotic or surgical drainage. The baby may have to be taken off the affected breast. She can feed from the other breast until treatment is completed.

The milk from the affected breast may be temporarily expressed and discarded. However, if the doctor feels that infection from the abscess is not present in the milk, he may not advise you to take the baby off the breast.

BABIES WITH PROBLEMS

FEEDING IN THE INCUBATOR

If the baby is put in an incubator for special care immediately after birth, and it is not allowed to come to you for feeds, express or pump your colostrum. Since it is very little in quantity, it can be fed to the baby by a nurse with the help of a spoon, dropper, tube, or drops fed from soaked gauze. Do not be dismayed if the amount of colostrum seems very little. The capacity of the baby's stomach is very small. A full-term newborn's stomach capacity on day one is 5 to 7 ml, that is, 1 to 1.4 teaspoonful. On day 3 it is 22 to 27 ml or 0.75 to 1 ounce. That is all the baby needs at one feed.

Even though the colostrum is very little in the beginning, each drop of it is worth its weight in gold, when you consider all the advantages it is going to give your baby. (See pg.127 COLOSTRUM)

Subsequently, breast milk should be expressed and given to the baby in the incubator. Or, better still, the mother can go to the nursery to suckle the baby at feed time.

Once colostrum has become milk, the best way to feed a baby is either

- via a tube
- directly from a stainless steel bowl or katori.
- or directly from the breast.

FEEDING LOW BIRTH WEIGHT & PREMATURE BABIES

Breast milk is the perfect food for low birth weight babies and babies born pre-term.

Low birth weight babies that are born weighing less than 2.5 kg at term and pre-term babies are those born earlier than 15 days before the estimated date of delivery. Breast milk of mothers of such babies has a higher concentration of protein, essential fatty acids and sodium which is more suitable for them.

When such babies are fed with breast milk it prevents them from having a drop in temperature, a drop in glucose levels and metabolic derangements. It also protects the baby from infection, enhances chances of survival and optimizes the baby's growth and development.

JAUNDICE

Jaundice is fairly common in babies. There are three kinds of jaundice, as explained below. Mostly, jaundice does not require treatment. It may require treatment if it occurs within 24 hours of birth. Jaundice needs treatment if the baby appears sick, drowsy, anaemic, or develops altered behaviour, a bleeding tendency, swelling of the body or persistent vomiting with dehydration.

KINDS OF JAUNDICE	TIME OF OCCURRENCE
Abnormal Jaundice	Occurs within 24 hours of birth. It needs urgent treatment in a hospital.
Physiological Jaundice	Occurs after 30 hours of birth, gradually deepens and disappears by the 10th day.
Breast Milk Jaundice	Starts at the end of the 1st week of life. It is at its worst during the 2nd and 3rd weeks. It can last upto 2 months.

ABNORMAL JAUNDICE

This kind of jaundice is today a thing of the past. An early pregnancy blood test identifies women with blood group incompatibility (see pg. 91 *"RHESUS NEGATIVE"*). Such women are given an anti-D immunoglobulin injection to prevent abnormal jaundice in the child. When this injection is not given, it results in blood group incompatibility.

Jaundice that occurs in the first 24 hours is more severe and serious and is called haemolytic jaundice. It may be the result of blood group incompatibility between the mother and the baby and needs urgent treatment to prevent brain damage in the child. The baby needs to be treated in a hospital. It may require complete blood transfusion, after which breastfeeding can continue normally.

However after the mother is given an injection of Anti-D immunoglobulin. She can safely feed the baby and the baby does not need a blood transfusion.

PHYSIOLOGICAL JAUNDICE

Physiological jaundice is fairly common, mild, and usually harmless. It occurs after 30 hours of birth, gradually deepens and disappears by the

10th day. The reason it happens is that within the uterus the baby has an abundance of red blood cells. Once the baby is born and breathing, an excessive amount of red blood cells is not needed, so they break down until the level of cells is appropriate for the baby. A byproduct of breakdown is bilirubin, which is normally expelled in the baby's first stool. Feeding of colostrum encourages this to happen. Feeding glucose water and other supplements does not help as they interfere with breastfeeding and can increase the possibility of jaundice.

According to Dr R. K. Anand, 'A rise of 0.5 mg./dl of bilirubin or more per hour or a falling haemoglobin level may need some intervention.

Children who are born normally without any problem are usually quite safe, but those who are born prematurely or had lack of oxygen, low blood sugar or accumulation of acids in the body (acidoses), need extra care.'

BREAST MILK JAUNDICE

This is a rare kind of jaundice that develops about a week after birth and could continue for 10 weeks. Although the jaundice may become as deep as 20 mg/dl bilirubin it does not harm the baby's brain, because it occurs after the first week of life, when the blood-brain barrier is well-developed. You can continue breastfeeding.

However, if your baby's bilirubin level rises too high, your paediatrician may request you to interrupt breastfeeding for a short while, say 12 hours or more. If at the end of this time the bilirubin level has fallen, it confirms that it has been caused by the presence of a harmless substance in breast milk. That is why it is referred to as 'breast milk jaundice'!

It is harmless, the baby gains weight normally and no treatment is required.

While your baby is off breast milk, keep your milk supply going by expression or pumping more frequently than your baby would have fed, and discard your milk until your milk can again be fed.

Generally jaundice is no cause to stop breastfeeding. Some people wrongly believe that breast milk jaundice means that breastfeeding should completely stop. This is not so. The condition resolves itself spontaneously in time with no ill-effects on the baby from breast milk.

Other causes of jaundice could be infection, metabolic conditions such as low blood sugar, or even administration of drugs to the mother in pregnancy.

TREATMENT

Babies with moderately raised levels of bilirubin are often treated by being placed uncovered in a cot 16 inches beneath a daylight fluorescent tube with their eyes covered. This is called phototherapy. There is no harm if you take the baby from under the light every 2 hours to feed, and maybe more often if the baby demands it. Remove the eye covers when you feed.

If your baby is otherwise well, your paediatrician may agree to your taking your baby home and giving it exposure to sunlight. You can place the baby in mild sunshine. Expose as much of the baby's body to sunlight as possible. Just make sure it does not get too hot or too cold. You can blindfold the baby

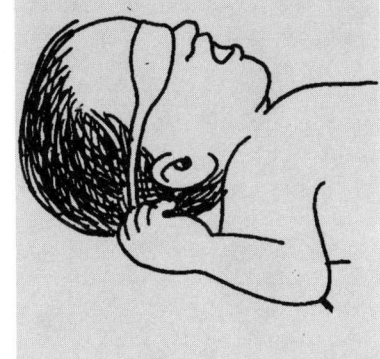

PHOTOTHERAPY

To treat high bilirubin levels the baby may be exposed to controlled amounts of ultra-violet light, which breaks down the pigment levels in the skin. The shades protect the eyes from the light.

if the sunlight is too strong, so that it does not affect the baby's eyesight. You may have to take your baby back to the hospital for blood tests.

CLEFT PALATE

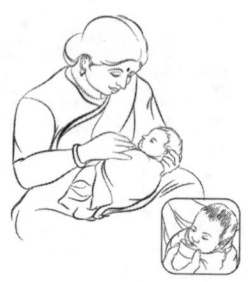

A cleft palate means that there is an opening on the roof of the baby's mouth. It might sometimes be accompanied by a cleft in the lip also. The cause of the cleft happens sometime within the first 3 months of the baby's development in the womb. There is not much you could have done about it, so do not add to your anxiety with your worry. Besides, do not let your relationship with your partner be tinged with unnecessary suspicion that the anomaly was caused by the other. Accept the baby and love it. Do not blame yourself.

A baby with a cleft lip & palate cannot suck. However it can cup feed. The baby must be cup feeding before palate repair surgery. Changing from bottle to cup post surgery can be upsetting for mother and baby. Therefore it is better to be cup feeding from the beginning.

HOW TO FEED A BABY BY CUP

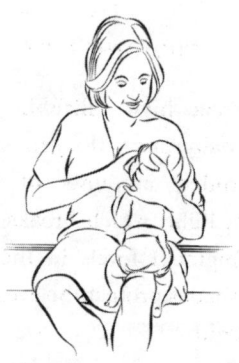

Hold the baby sitting upright or semi-upright on your lap. Hold the small cup of milk to the baby's lips, by resting it on baby's lower lip. Tilt cup so that the milk reaches the baby's upper lip.

The baby becomes alert. The baby starts to take the milk into his mouth with his tongue. Do not pour the milk into the baby's mouth. Just hold the cup to his lips and let him take it himself.

When the baby has had enough, he closes his mouth and will not take any more. If he has not taken the calculated amount, he may take more next time, or you may need to feed him more often.

A full term or older baby sucks the milk, spilling some of it.

Measure his intake over 24 hours not just at each feed.

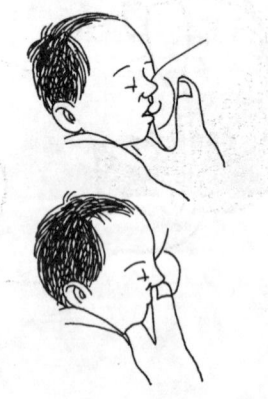

Provide a nurturing environment when cup feeding. Give baby a soft blanket or toy to hold. Hold the baby close to you in a comfortable position for baby. Speak softly with baby and do not rush him.

Breastfeeding a baby with a cleft palate can be difficult. The baby needs to attach itself properly to the breast so that it can suck well. The best position at the breast for a baby with a cleft palate is one with the nose and throat higher than the breast. The upright position is therefore very good.

The baby's body should be in an upright position close to the mother's. This position will prevent milk from leaking through the opening on the roof of the baby's mouth into the nose. If milk does go into the baby's nose, it makes it difficult for the baby to breathe. When the baby is well attached to the breast, the breast tissue closes over the cleft and helps the baby suck well.

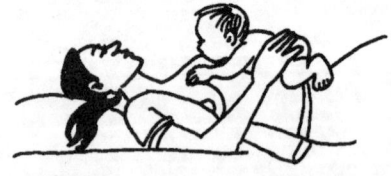

Babies with a cleft palate have a tendency for their tongue to fall back. So another good position for feeding such a baby is with the mother lying on her back and the baby lying on top of her for feeding. This position ensures that the baby's tongue remains forward, thus making it possible for the baby to suck well.

Apart from the above positions, the mother can also express milk and feed it with a spoon to the baby placed on her lap with the head held higher than the rest of the body.

The baby will have to be fed thus until the condition can be rectified by surgery. Generally 2 or 3 surgeries will be required. Apart from the paediatrician, the parents will also have to consult a plastic surgeon, a dentist, a prosthodontist, and maybe a speech therapist.

As suggested by a leading paediatrician, a dentist (prosthodontist) may be consulted to fit the baby with an artificial palate to cover the gap on the roof of the baby's mouth, so that the baby can be breastfed. Some doctors fear that the artificial palate might cause infection at the site. But with breast milk the baby will receive infection-fighting properties and put on weight. Besides, any wound arising from the procedure will heal really quickly in a day or two, since it is in the mouth, an area where healing is quick.

Whether the mother nurses the baby at the breast, or with a spoon, she should cuddle the baby and keep trying to nurse it at the breast. Such non-nutritive suckling helps mother and baby bond to each other.

A cleft palate and/or lip must be operated within a year, before the baby starts to speak. Sometimes a baby with a cleft palate may be more prone to ear infections.

This condition requires an enormous amount of patience on the part of the parents. However, one day, all of your efforts will be behind you and your baby's condition will stand corrected with no cosmetic and functional problem. At the present moment, if your baby does have this problem, it will help immensely if you can be in touch with a couple who has gone through a similar experience recently. It may be someone distantly related or an acquaintance. Search them out for they can be beacons of moral support to you. If you do not know anyone, or meet someone who is not forthcoming, ask your paediatrician or plastic surgeon.

16

AFTER CHILDBIRTH

IMMEDIATELY AFTER THE birth of the baby you may not be overcome by a gush of maternal love and instincts. You might even be a little disappointed by the way your baby looks. This is quite normal. As you begin to breastfeed and care for your baby, as you see your baby respond to you, your maternal feelings will be aroused and a deep love for your baby will bloom.

It is a good idea to take a laxative tablet after the birth of the baby so that you can pass the first stool with ease. Other tablets that may be prescribed by your doctor could be antibiotics for your stitches, pain-killers, or tablets for bleeding.

After the birth of the baby, and always afterwards, do not wash yourself from the anus towards the vagina after passing a stool. You could infect your stitches and make them septic, or cause yourself a urinary tract infection. Wash the anal area separately with soap, after passing a stool.

AFTER A NORMAL BIRTH

After normal vaginal delivery of the baby, you may find that you have to contend with discomfort in some parts of your body. Your breasts, for instance, a few days after birth, would become full/swollen/sensitive as the milk comes in. Pressing out some milk when this happens will help relieve the discomfort. Sometimes you might experience mild contractions while feeding, for, as you feed, hormones are released that contract the uterus and encourage it to involute close to its pre-pregnant size. Practise waist-level breathing to get over this discomfort.

Your perineum or pelvic floor may be sore from the stitches, so for the first 4 to 5 days sitting may be a problem. It will help if you use a round rubber tube to sit upon, like the one children use in swimming pools. It will avoid direct pressure on the perineum when you are sitting, so healing will be quick and the discomfort less; specially when you sit up to breastfeed the baby. Alternatively, you could sit between two pillows.

If during your bath you bathe the vaginal area and the perineum with a mug of warm water to which a few drops, 8 or 10, of the homoeopathic medicine calendula Q have been added, the healing will be much faster. The doctor will give you an ointment to apply, a mycin, and perhaps an anesthetic ointment.

Your stomach will feel jelly-like, loose and unstable. You must exercise

PRECAUTION

If you bend forward when passing urine you prevent it dribbling backwards towards the vagina/vaginal stitches. This prevents infection.

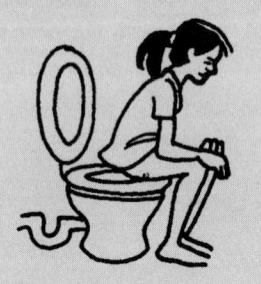

your abdominal muscles in the first few weeks to regain abdominal tone. *(See postnatal exercises below.)*

Avoid wearing a corset or binding cloth around your abdomen. It will only get your muscles used to artificial support. The minute the support is removed, the muscles will sag.

Immediately after birth the muscles are still under the influence of relaxing hormones. The exercises you do should merely coax the muscles back to their original position from their stretched positions. Special exercises are needed for this. Avoid squatting exercises. Do not lift both legs together when lying on your back. It will cause great strain on the lower back. Do not cycle in the air.

Since your muscles are in a relaxed state and your body, especially your back, has been overstrained, get extra help to take care of household chores for this period so that you can rest and concentrate on breastfeeding the baby.

When you work, say, when you wash or iron, make sure that you do so without unnecessary exertion. That is, sit comfortably on a low stool when you wash the diapers. Make sure the ironing surface is the correct height for you. You should not have to bend when you iron, or, push the baby's pram, or cook. Keep your elbows relaxed and do not tense your shoulders. Overstrain, when performing simple day-to-day tasks, can give rise to discomfort or pain in some of the muscles in your body. If you are unlucky, this pain might stay with you even later; so make sure you do not overstrain. Do not lift anything heavy. When lifting anything of moderate weight, bend knees and keep the back straight as you do so. Whenever you bend down to make the bed or pick up something you may have dropped, pull in your abdomen first.

Your lower abdomen may be streaked with brown or purple lines. These lines will slowly fade to white and become less prominent. They are called stretch marks and tend to stay, getting fainter over the years.

At times you may be troubled with piles after childbirth. You might feel itchy around the anus. When piles are greatly aggravated they may even bleed. If you splash the anal area with cold water and then dab it dry, it will relieve the itching. Avoid spicy foods. A number of women have found the internal and external application of the ointment Procto Sedyl very comforting.

One can also take a medicine available at a homoeopathic pharmacy called Bio-combination number 17 as per instructions on the bottle. One can have it for approximately a month or until the piles are resolved. For some women that could mean 2 to 3 months.

You must make sure you do pelvic floor exercises as described in the postnatal exercises, so that you regain the tone of those muscles and do not end up losing control of passing urine, or slackening of these muscles.

Although you will lose some weight at birth, it will take some time to regain your figure. Give yourself 8 months to a year. If you are considerably overweight you will have to work at it. At birth your weight loss will be equivalent to the weight of the placenta, the baby and the amniotic fluid. Over the weeks following the birth you will lose a lot of the extra fluid content of your body.

Changing baby's diaper

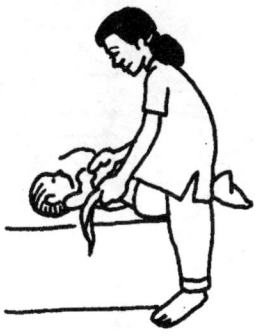

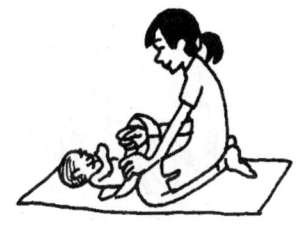

Tackling household chores

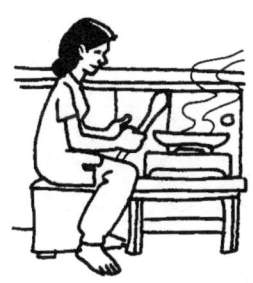

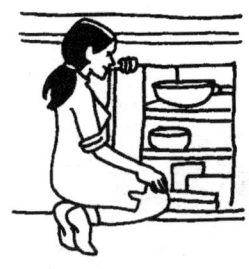

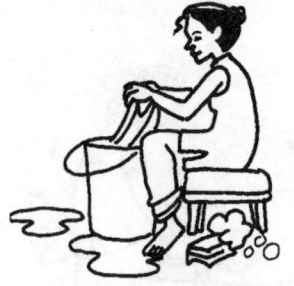

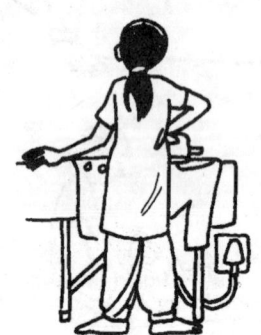

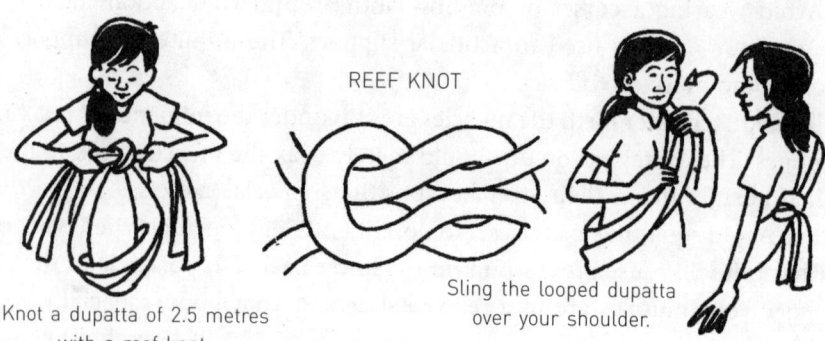

A SLING FOR THE BABY

REEF KNOT

Knot a dupatta of 2.5 metres with a reef knot.

Sling the looped dupatta over your shoulder.

It will look like this from the back

Push the cloth inside out to make a sling for the baby.

Place the baby in the sling. You now have both hands free to work with.

Older babies can be made to sit in the sling

EXERCISES AFTER A NORMAL DELIVERY

When you lie down to exercise, always do so without a pillow.

Days 1 & 2
Exercise 1
Lie on your back with knees bent, feet resting on the bed. Breathe in slowly and deeply, breathe out. Do this every day, between each exercise and at the end.
   Do 5 times.

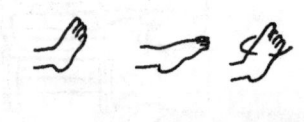
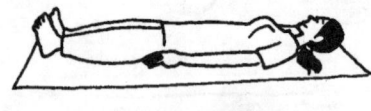

Exercise 2
Lie with your legs straight and slightly apart. Bend and stretch your toes. Bend and stretch your ankles. Roll your feet in circles in both directions. Do 5 times in each direction.
   Repeat this 5 times.

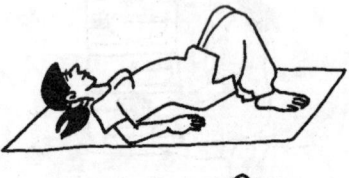

Exercise 3
Lie on your back with knees bent and feet resting on the bed. Tighten your buttock muscles and pull in your abdomen so that your back is pressed against the bed. Hold this position while you count to 6, then relax. Take

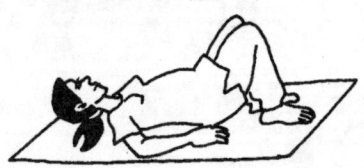

two normal breaths, then exhale and repeat.
   Do 5 times.

Day 3
Repeat the above exercises and add exercise 4, which will strengthen the muscles supporting the womb and help keep it in its correct position.

Exercise 4
This can be done sitting or lying down. Exhale, pull up the muscles through which your baby was born, thus tightening your vaginal muscles, i.e. you contract just as you would when you try to stop the flow of urine. Hold the contraction while you count 6; then relax. Exhale. Repeat.
   Do 5 times, always exhaling before you start.

Days 4 to 7
Exercise 5
Lie with your right knee bent, and right foot on bed, left leg straight. Slide your straight leg (left) down the bed, as far as possible, then slide the whole leg up the bed.
   Only your waist muscles must work. Repeat with the other leg.
   Do 4 times with each leg.

Exercise 6
Lie with knees bent and feet on bed.
Draw in your abdominal muscles, reach across your body to place one hand on the opposite side of the bed, level with your hips. Return to the starting position. Now do this with the other hand. Do 8 times.
   In the afternoon sleep on your stomach. Put a pillow under your head and one below your breasts to avoid discomfort.

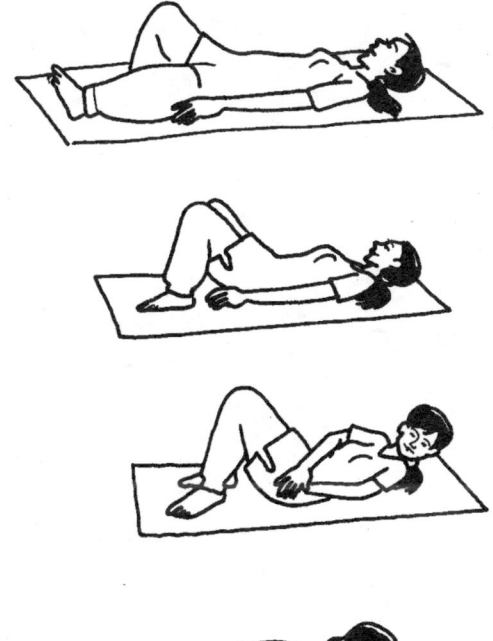

AFTER A CAESAREAN SECTION

After the birth of your baby by abdominal surgery, with general anesthesia, the first thing to strike you could be the discomfort of your abdominal scar. You would then be introduced to your baby. If you do some deep breathing (waist-level), as much as you can comfortably manage, it will help to exhale the anesthesia out of your tissues and make you feel better.

   In case of a Caesarean delivery by epidural/spinal anesthesia you could ask to have your baby placed on you immediately. You could place the baby on your chest diagonally or have it placed over your shoulder, with head towards your breast and feet towards your shoulder. As the effect of the epidural/spinal anesthesia wears off, discomfort may be felt. Do the waist-level breathing or any other labour breathing to help you cope.

   It is common after surgery with general anesthesia to feel that you have a collection of mucus in your throat. Some women say, 'I have just developed a bad throat.' The discomfort in the throat is caused as a result of a rubber tube inserted in your windpipe during surgery, so that if you vomit while under anesthesia you do not inhale it into your lungs. It may cause a lot of dryness in the throat and make you want to cough. If you feel dryness in your throat, cover your mouth with a wet towel as you breathe, and/or put a couple of drops of water in your mouth to prevent dryness. When dryness does not bother you any longer, suck some cough drops or rock sugar (mishri) to soothe the throat.

However, now, there is an improvement in the techniques used, as a result of which post-operative discomfort is a lot less.

The sooner you cough up the phlegm from your throat, the better you will feel. You have to learn to cough in your throat like singers before a vocal recital. Clear your throat and cough out. This will be more effective than taking cough syrup. The sooner the throat gets cleared, the better you will feel. Practise coughing in your throat rather than from your abdomen, just so that you can do it easily if ever required.

The internal stitches on your abdomen will dissolve, but the external stitches may need to be removed a week to 10 days later. On the other hand, the external stitches may also be the dissolving kind. You will have to take it easy to allow the healing to take place.

On the 2nd day the nurse will come to change the sheets of your bed. It will be better if you get out of bed while she does so. Sit up in bed, by having your bed shifted to a sitting position. Place palms on either side of your body and lift your body up and gradually move yourself to the edge of the bed. Gently swing legs off the bed on the footstool or floor, hold a pillow in front of the abdomen for support, stand up and move to sit on a sofa/chair. Go back gently to the bed when it is made. The whole exercise will make you feel much better by the end of it, since it will give an impetus to your blood circulation.

If your first delivery is by a Caesarean section for a non-recurring factor like failed induction or fetal distress, then the second delivery could be a normal delivery.

If the first delivery is by Caesarean section for a recurring factor like a malformed pelvis, then the second delivery will also be by Caesarean section. (*Read the section on vaginal birth after caesarean section, VBAC.*)

EXERCISES BEFORE STITCHES ARE REMOVED

The following are gentle exercises to be done after a Caesarean section.

Exercise 1
Lie on your back. Breathe in slowly and deeply, breathe out. Do 5 times, at least twice a day.

Exercise 2
Lie with your legs straight and slightly apart. Bend and stretch your ankles. Bend and stretch your toes. Roll your feet in circles in both directions. (*See above.*)

Exercise 3
This exercise can be done sitting or lying down. Exhale, pull up the muscles of the pelvic floor, thus tightening your vaginal muscles, i.e. you contract just like you would when you try to stop the flow of urine. Hold the contraction as you count to 6, then relax. Exhale. Repeat. Do 5 times, always exhaling before you start. *(see above)*

EXERCISES AFTER REMOVAL OF STITCHES

Exercises after the removal of the stitches on the 7th and 8th day after a Caesarean section and after 7/8 days after a normal delivery when you are up and about all day.

Exercise 1
Stand with legs crossed at ankles, press thighs, contract between the legs as you would when you try to stop the flow of urine, pull in the abdomen and also tighten buttocks and anus. Hold it all tight for a count of 4, then relax. Repeat 6 times, always exhaling before you start.

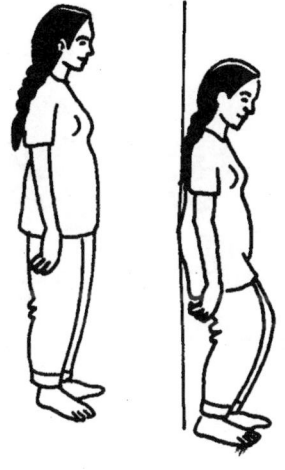

Exercise 2
Stand with your back against the wall. Tighten buttock muscles and pull in the abdominal wall and try to get the lower part of your back and your entire backbone to touch the wall. (This exercise can also be done lying on the bed, same as Exercise 3, after a normal delivery.)
Repeat 6 times, always exhaling before you start.

Exercise 3
Standing, pull one leg up at the hip so that one leg is shorter than the other. Keep the knee straight as you do this, and lift foot off the ground.
Repeat with the other leg.
Do 4 times, and build up to 8 times. (Can also be done lying down as in Exercise 5 after a normal delivery.)

Exercise 4
Stand with feet together, knees together, thighs pressed together. Move along the floor as if twisting for a short distance. Do once.
These simple exercises done for the first 40 days will do your figure miles and miles of good which even strenuous workouts later will not be able to achieve.

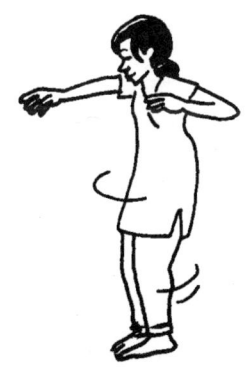

Exercise 5
After breastfeeding is completed, or when breast feeding is minimal towards the end, say 2 or 3 feeds a day, do the bust exercise. (*see Bust Exercise in the chapter, Some Simple Exercises.*) Earlier than that, when breastfeeding exclusively, you can do Section B of the bust exercise.

BLEEDING/SEX

After the birth of the baby vaginally or after a Caesarean section you will have a longish period lasting a week or several weeks (maybe 4 to 6 weeks). Thereafter you may not have a period for several months, especially if you are breastfeeding exclusively.

The first period that occurs is usually longer and heavier than a normal period. It could last 7 days or more. Thereafter your regular cycle will set in. When the first period occurs is totally unpredictable. With breastfeeding it could come after 3 to 4 months, or after 6 to 9 months. In women who do not breastfeed, the period could start on the 28th day after the birth of the baby. The post-delivery discharge could be brownish/pinkish/occasionally red (when exertion is undertaken).

Not having a period need not mean that you are pregnant. Neither does it mean that since you are not getting a period you cannot become pregnant. You must use some contraceptive in consultation with your doctor. As soon as you feel you have healed vaginally, you can resume intercourse. This might take 10 days or so. Some women like to wait up to 40 days or 6 weeks. You can use some lubricant like petroleum jelly if required.

When you go to the doctor for a check-up you must inform him or her of any discomfort you might have with your bowel movement, passing of urine, sexual intercourse, or piles. Pelvic or pelvic floor discomfort would also need investigation.

You may walk up and down the stairs, but not more than is absolutely essential, that is, keep it to a minimum. Get as much rest as possible. Sleep for 2 hours in the afternoon. Go back to bed after the early morning feed at 5 or 6 a.m.

POST-NATAL DEPRESSION

It is common to have mood swings after the birth of the baby. Some women feel positive while others might feel negative.

When a woman is overly depressed, it is called post-partum psychosis. A woman suffering from post-partum depression will cry easily, sleep with difficulty, be tired and irritable, experience fear or a feeling of inferiority or inadequacy.

At times a woman feels resentful that from being a pampered pregnant woman she is now a responsible mother. Depression may also creep in when you feel depressed about the kind of birth experience you have had, or when you are overburdened with work and have no help to tide over this physically taxing phase in your life.

Occasionally, the reality of babycare might be overwhelming. One mother helplessly exclaimed, 'But my baby smells shitty and vomity.' Your baby simply does not look and smell like the advertisements suggest. It will be better if you do not discuss your feelings with unsympathetic persons. But do discuss them with a trusted friend. It is healthy not to bottle up these negative emotions. Take things easy, do not worry too much about housework. There is no harm if household chores go unattended for a short while.

If depression persists consult a sympathetic doctor, whether your family physician or a homoeopathic doctor. Alternatively, you can consult a psychologist or psychotherapist. Discussing your feelings with them will help tremendously in removing a psychological knot in your mind and unblock a lot of energy, so that you will feel and function better.

Depression can occur in a perfectly healthy woman. It might be caused by a sudden withdrawal of hormones from your body after the birth of the baby. The doctor might prescribe some artificial hormones for a while, the dosage of which he will gradually taper off. Alternatively, the doctor may prescribe anti-depressant drugs. Most women have responded very well to homoeopathic medicines. In case postnatal depression does occur, women who take homoeopathic medicines tide over it quickly and effectively.

17 CONTRACEPTION

IN ORDER TO understand contraception it is important to understand how pregnancy takes place. For pregnancy to take place, an ovum or egg is released by one of the ovaries in the woman's body. When it is fertilized by a sperm, pregnancy begins. The release of the ovum in the woman's body is called ovulation.

Sperm is contained in the semi-gelatinous seminal fluid of the male ejaculation, which is slightly alkaline. Unless sperm gains access to the mouth of the womb or the cervix within 15 to 20 minutes following ejaculation, it is killed by the acid medium of the vagina. The cervix has an alkaline environment, so that sperm rapidly swims through it, up into the womb, and past the womb, along the fallopian tubes. In the fallopian tubes the ovum is fertilized. This journey takes 45 minutes. Sperm can survive and fertilize the ovum for approximately 2 days. Sometimes sperm cells can survive for 7 days. After being fertilised, the ovum takes 7 days to travel the length of the fallopian tube and reach the womb or uterus.

ABSTINENCE

The only sure way of not conceiving is to avoid intercourse altogether. However, this may be quite bad for your relationship with your husband.

COITUS INTERRUPTUS OR THE WITHDRAWAL METHOD

It is a method in which the penis is withdrawn before ejaculation. It requires a great amount of self-control by the man. Besides, sperm is present even in the leakage preceding ejaculation, and, from the region of the vulva where it may be deposited it can enter the vagina even when penetration does not take place. From the vagina it can enter the uterus and end up fertilizing an ovum, leading to pregnancy. This is therefore a very unreliable method and should not be depended upon.

RHYTHM METHOD

This is a natural method of birth control. For it to be successful it is important to pinpoint the time of ovulation, that is, the release of the ovum by the ovary, and its subsequent fertilization. Ovulation generally occurs 14 days before the onset of the next period. If the ovum is not fertilized in approximately 18 hours it dies.

The first requirement of the use of this method is a regular cycle of periods occurring at regular and fixed intervals. The next step is to pinpoint the 14th day before the next cycle. If the periods occur at irregular intervals, it will be difficult to pinpoint this day. The exact timing of ovulation may vary slightly.

Sometimes shock, tension, or strain can further interfere with ovulation, causing it to occur anywhere from the 11th to the 17th day before the next cycle. Also, a perfectly predictable menstrual cycle may become irregular as a result of travel, strain, illness, in the late 30s or early 40s, or after childbirth. During such times the method is unreliable.

In a regular 28-day cycle, it is not possible for conception to occur in the first 8 days of the menstrual cycle, beginning from the first day of the onset of the menstrual bleeding. So if there are 5 days of bleeding, 3 days after the bleeding are safe. Then the fertile period would be from the 9th to the 17th day, both days inclusive. From the 18th to the 28th day would again be a safe period.

In a woman with a 35-day cycle, the fertile period would be from the 15th to the 25th day, both days inclusive.

The rhythm method presupposes a perfectly regular cycle.

Another pitfall of the rhythm method is that occasionally, ovulation may be provoked by sexual stimulation, regardless of the time of the fertile or non-fertile phase of the menstrual cycle.

Some lucky women find that this method works for them. They are very strict with their calculations and self-control. It may be a problem for women whose husbands tour a lot and happen to be home on the wrong days of the month. Besides, it does not always work.

Added to the rhythm method, for greater accuracy one can follow the temperature method. Before ovulation a woman's body temperature dips slightly and when ovulation occurs, it rises slightly. A dip in the temperature signifies that the ovum is ready for release. A rise signifies the release of the ovum.

TEMPERATURE METHOD

The temperature dips by just about 1 degree below the normal body temperature, and rises by just 1 degree above the normal body temperature on the Fahrenheit thermometer. It rises half a degree on the Centigrade thermometer scale. The temperature should therefore be taken by a very sensitive thermometer. After rising, the temperature remains high for 2 weeks, until the next period begins. A daily record has to be kept. It has to be tried for at least 6 months in order to be understood and followed accurately. If you are suffering from a fever or infection, the temperature reading will not be accurate.

The temperature has to be taken at the same time every day. It has to be taken when you wake up in the morning, before getting out of bed and before taking food and drink. The thermometer must be left in place for at least 3 minutes.

The temperature reading could vary according to your menstrual cycle, the shortest cycle being 21 days and the longest 45 days. In a 28-day cycle the temperature would rise on approximately the 14th day after the first day of the menstrual period. In a 37-day cycle the temperature would rise on the 22nd day after the first day of the menstrual period.

If your temperature reading does not show the kind of reading mentioned here, continue to keep the record nevertheless. It would be of interest to your doctor as and when you go for consultations.

CHECKING THE CERVICAL MUCUS OR THE BILLINGS METHOD

Vaginal secretions change during your cycle. A few days after your menstrual period you may notice a thick, cloudy and sticky mucus secretion. Around the time of ovulation it will change to clear, stretchy and abundant mucus. This attracts the sperm and allows easy penetration of it to fertilize the ovum. After the fertility period is over, the mucus again becomes thick, gelatinous and hostile to sperm.

To test vaginal secretions, you must first wash your hands with soap, then insert your finger in the vagina in order to get a sample of the secretion. Notice the nature of the secretion. It will take you a few months to accurately understand the secretions. Besides, sometimes semen may mask the true nature of your vaginal secretions. This method is also undesirable because it can cause vaginal infection and the mucus secretions cannot be accurately interpreted by the layman.

BREASTFEEDING

If your baby is 100% breastfed, it will change the levels of hormones in your body and prevent ovulation. That is, if you are demand-feeding your baby with no complementary bottles or other foods, a high level of prolactin hormone in your body will suppress ovulation. Breastfeeding also delays the onset of your next period. If you breastfeed on demand in the first few months, your period can take 6 to 8 months to return. If you add complementary bottles and other foods to the baby's diet, your period could return in 2 to 4 months. On the other hand, when breastfeeding is continued unrestrictedly, your periods may take a year or more to return.

Even when you do not have a period, you could ovulate and become pregnant. On the other hand, some women may have a period or two that may be anovular, that is, not accompanied by ovulation, or a release of the egg. Hence, breastfeeding and menstruation are unreliable indexes to whether you can conceive or not.

Along with breastfeeding, if you take the progestogen-only pill or the mini-pill it will help prevent conception, since it will be combined with reduced fertility produced by breastfeeding. You should not have the regular oestrogen-progestogen combined pill, since it will reduce milk production and have other undesirable side-effects. When you go for a check-up 6 weeks after delivery, tell the doctor you are breastfeeding and ask for advice. If you have intercourse before the 6-week period, you must use some other contraceptive, for instance, the condom.

The pill has one disadvantage. Its hormones are secreted in the milk and studies are continuing to find out if they have any ill-effects on the baby. If you find that after taking the pill your baby has become irritable and is not gaining weight as before, go off the pill and try some other contraceptive.

A breastfeeding woman should start the pill about 21 days before she plans to start weaning her baby with supplementary foods. If her period does not occur after the first course of tablets, she should wait 7 days and start the next course of tablets. A period will occur after weaning has been completed.

PILLS

Pills are made of a combination of the 2 hormones, oestrogen and progestogen. The modern contraceptive pill has approximately 10% of the dose of hormones as compared to the pill in use 20 years ago. As a result, the side-effects are fewer and less severe. The hormones in the pill suppress the production of eggs by the ovaries by fooling them into believing that you are already pregnant. The pill is easily available in the market under different brand names.

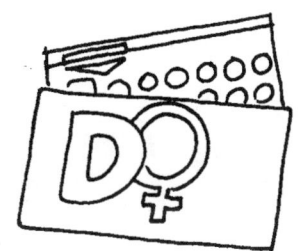

Since the hormonal dosage is greatly reduced, breakthrough bleeding sometimes occurs as a result of hormonal imbalance. In the first few days or the first few cycles of taking the pill, bleeding occurs. The blood loss usually occurs around the 17th day of the cycle and continues for a few days or until the next period. It appears in the form of spotting. The pills should be continued nevertheless. However, if it recurs, inform your doctor. It is possible that the doctor will change it to a pill with a higher hormone level to prevent further bleeding.

The pill should not be taken by young women whose bone growth is still not completed and who have not yet reached physical maturity. It should also be avoided by women above 35 years of age, women who smoke, those who have suffered from malignant disease, liver dysfunction, cardiac disease, kidney disease, diabetes, depression, epilepsy, or those having a previous history of thromboembolic manifestations or thrombophlebitis (problems with the clotting of the blood), bronchial asthma, or migraine.

When taken, it is important that it is taken at the same time every day. Its advantage is that it is the most efficient means of contraception. The failure rate is nil. It does not interfere with the spontaneity of sexual intercourse, and does not involve any mechanical device. It controls the menstrual cycle to 28 days, and reduces the amount of menstrual flow. It also eliminates or controls menstrual pain.

Just as some people are sensitive to certain drugs, e.g. some kinds of antibiotics, in the same way some women are sensitive to the pill. The possible side-effects of the pill are nausea, fluid retention, weight gain, enlarged and painful breasts, change in sexual desire, or fungal infection in the vagina. Should any of these symptoms arise, you can discuss with your doctor whether you want to continue with the pill or switch to another contraceptive.

If on the pill, it is a good idea to take a break from it every 6 months. For 2 months use some other contraceptive and then get back to the pill. Allow 2 to 3 months to pass before becoming pregnant, so that you are sure that all the hormones have passed out of your system before you conceive. You will also be able to date your pregnancy more accurately.

The pill reduces the level of Vitamin B_6, folic acid, calcium, manganese, zinc and ascorbic acid in your body. It is therefore a good idea to take multi-vitamins along with it.

THE INTRA-UTERINE DEVICE (IUD)

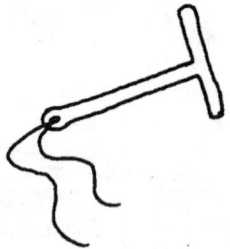

Cooper T

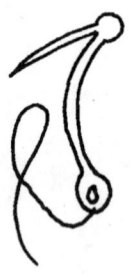

Cooper 7

The intra-uterine device is a tiny device with a copper coil that can be inserted into the uterus during a vaginal examination, and left there. It can be inserted 6 weeks after the birth of the baby, after a normal delivery. The copper in this device makes the cervical mucus thick. Copper also makes the uterine lining hostile to the implantation of the fertilized ovum. Although the success rate with the IUD is high, it is not 100 percent reliable, since it is only a mechanical hindrance to pregnancy. Should pregnancy occur and you decide to keep it, the IUD will be left inside. There is the possibility that the IUD may not be there at all. That is, you might have lost it, without realizing it. If it is there, it can get embedded in the placenta, and be delivered with it after the birth of the baby or discharged with the period-like discharge after the birth of the baby. Should you decide to go for a medical termination of pregnancy, it should definitely be done within 12 weeks, or, maximum before 20 weeks after the 1st day of the last menstrual period. During the abortion, the IUD will also be removed.

There are various brands of IUDs available such as Copper T, the Copper-7, and the Mutiload. If the insertion of the IUD does not suit a woman, that is, if it gives rise to profuse bleeding or pain, it can be removed and then re-inserted after 2 to 3 months. The first few periods after its insertion may be heavy. This may not matter in some cases. However, if a woman already has heavy periods or is anaemic, it may not be advisable.

It is not advisable for a woman who has not had any children to use an IUD. IUDs have been known to cause perforation of the uterus, septic abortion, pelvic inflammation and ectopic pregnancy. Women with fibroids in the uterus or a prolapsed uterus should also avoid the IUD.

In the case of a normal delivery it can be inserted after 6 weeks (3 months after a Caesarean delivery). Otherwise it is preferable to insert it 2 to 3 days after the period is over. It could also be inserted during a period, or 6 weeks after a medically carried out or natural abortion.

After insertion it will give you a 2-to-3-year holiday from contraception worries since that is how long it will remain effective. It is therefore a good device to be used between pregnancies, to space children. If pregnancy is desired before that period, it can be removed as easily as it is inserted. It does not interfere with breastfeeding, nor does it introduce hormones into a woman's body. It can be removed as and when another pregnancy is desired.

A woman who has had an IUD inserted must make sure she has it removed after its effectiveness has dissipated. Your doctor will tell you when that will be.

CONDOM

The condom is a rubber sheath that is placed over the erect penis before penetration. It works by preventing the sperm from entering the vagina. Various kinds are available in the market under different brand names. If it is lubricated and freed of air before use, it is less likely to burst inside the vagina.

Sometimes it is not very effective because sperm may be deposited on the vulva before it is put on, through mild leaking from the penis that may take place earlier. Its efficacy depends on the care with which it is used. Use with a soluble spermicidal pessary in the vagina can greatly reduce its failure rate.

Some men do not like the condom as it takes away part of the sensation or because of the interference it brings into lovemaking, taking away spontaneity. However, used with care along with vaginal pessaries when other contraceptive methods are not available, it is very valuable. It also reduces the chances of catching sexually transmitted diseases, including the deadly disease, AIDS.

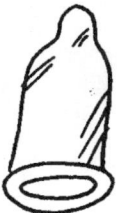
Confom

DIAPHRAGM OR THE CERVICAL CAP

These are cones made of rubber with metal at the rim.

They are fitted by the woman inside her body, in the vagina, over the cervix before intercourse and kept inside for 6 to 8 hours after intercourse. Along with them spermicidal creams have to be used. They have to be fitted by medical personnel for the correct size, and kept clean to avoid infection.

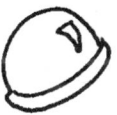

SPERMICIDAL PESSARIES

Spermicidal pessaries should be inserted into the vagina at least 4 to 5 minutes before intercourse. The contraceptive effect lasts for upto 1 hour. It can be used by itself, or together with the condom. It is more effective when used with the condom, since it must be at the cervix, not only somewhere in the vagina, when the sperm reaches the cervix or the mouth of the womb. The manufacturer's instructions should be followed carefully.

MORNING-AFTER CONTRACEPTION

This method should not be resorted to regularly. It is only to be used in emergencies. High dose morning—after pills can be had from a doctor or a family planning clinic. The pills are the ordinary combined oestrogen-progestogen contraceptive pills, not the mini-pill. A woman should take 2 of these pills as soon as possible and another 2.5 hours later. These pills have to be taken within 72 hours or 3 days of the intercourse. There is generally nausea and vomiting after it. Some women might also experience headache, dizziness, and tender breasts.

IUD AS EMERGENCY CONTRACEPTION

An IUD (intra-uterine device) fitted up to 7 days after sexual intercourse can prevent implantation of the fertilised egg in the womb. Although this will prevent a pregnancy, women often complain of a lot of pain and some bleeding.

SURGICAL STERILIZATION: FEMALE

Surgical sterilization of the female is called tubal ligation or tubectomy. During the operation the fallopian tubes which carry the egg from the ovary to the womb are tied and cut, or alternatively rings and clips are fixed on the fallopian tubes to block the passage of the egg from the ovary to the womb. It requires general anesthesia and a stay at the hospital for 2 to 3 days. If you have rings or clips on the fallopian tubes, the operation is more easily reversible. However, when getting it done, one should consider it as being irreversible. If during the operation the tubes get injured and bleed uncontrollably, they would be cut. When the tubes are cut or removed, reconstruction in order to make the surgery reversible will be impossible. Careful thought should be given before getting it done.

Apart from convalescence after the operation, it has no side-effects. Periods, intercourse, menopause and sexual desire remain unchanged. In very rare cases women have been known to become pregnant after this surgery.

SURGICAL STERILIZATION: MALE

Surgical sterilization of the male is called vasectomy. It is a simple operation. The tubes which carry the sperm from the testes to the penis are cut and tied. It is a minor surgery needing 15 to 30 minutes and can be carried out under a local anesthetic. If it is carried out under a general anesthetic the patient will need to stay in the hospital for a day.

It is a much simpler operation as compared with female sterilization. It has the further advantage of being reversible in 70% of cases. However, like female sterilization, it should be regarded as irreversible.

After the operation there are no side-effects, no change in sexual desire, strength or intercourse. If the man feels any change of sexual feelings, the problem is purely psychological. The man ejaculates as before, only the fluid will not contain any sperm. Following a vasectomy, sperm is still present in seminal fluid for some weeks. Contraception has to be used until the seminal fluid becomes sperm-free. This would require seminal analysis. When 2 consecutive analyses show an absence of sperm cells, only then can a man indulge in contraceptive-free intercourse.

MEDICINE FOR ABORTION

Recently, the government has approved a medicine for abortion. It has to be taken within 49 days or 7 weeks of pregnancy, that is, about 19 to 20 days after a missed period. Before the medicine is given, the doctor will check and rule out an ectopic pregnancy. The medicine is made up of two drugs, one is an anti-pregnancy (anti-progesterone) drug and the other is an expulsive drug (prostaglandin). After it is given, bleeding starts and can continue for 7 to 10 days. After the bleeding stops, an ultrasound is done to make sure abortion is complete. In case of an incomplete abortion, a minor operation (D&C) will be performed. This medicine therefore can be used only where medical support and back-up are available. It has a 95% success rate. In 5% of cases when it fails, it has to be backed up by a D&C.

CONTRACEPTION IN THE FUTURE

Various methods of contraception are currently being researched. However, no ideal solution has yet been found.

At present, research is taking place on vaccines or injections to prevent pregnancies; also on hormone implants under the skin in women for contraceptive purposes; on hormone preparations that can be taken like snuff; on better-quality condoms; on effective methods of pinpointing ovulation precisely, to help those who would like to use the rhythm method. The male pill has been tried and found to have too many negative side-effects. There is also research on surgical insertion of a valve in the tubes of the man and woman, to be removed as required at a later date. Who knows what course future contraception will take?

18

CONDITIONS THAT MAY REQUIRE SURGERY AT BIRTH

WHEN THE BABY is born there is a lot of excitement and a sigh of relief at the birth. The mother is tired but happy. The baby is looked at by the attending doctor, and now in most major centres and hospitals the delivery is attended by a paediatrician who examines the baby for normal reflexes and to check that the baby is breathing normally and has no obvious congenital anomalies.

It is increasingly becoming common to have antenatally diagnosed surgical conditions of which the parents are already aware. When such a situation arises it is imperative that the parents be in touch with a paediatric surgeon who will counsel them about the problem. This is important, as often the problem is completely curable and rarely is it life-threatening. Either way, it is good for the family to be mentally prepared.

There are a few conditions that alert the doctor to the immediate need for surgery on the baby:

Gastroschisis
The intestines are lying outside the abdomen through an opening in the abdomen.

Omphalocoel
A sac is covering the extruded intestines.

Oesophageal Atresia & Tracheo-Oesophageal Fistula
The baby has increased frothing at the mouth and is unable to accept feeds, due to a communication between the air pipe (trachea) and food pipe (oesophagus).

Diaphragmatic Hernia
The baby has breathing difficulty. The abdomen is flattened and the intestines and liver are lying in the chest and are detected clinically by hearing bowel sounds in the chest and plain X-ray of the chest reveals bowel shadows in the chest.

Imperforate anus
There is no anal opening.

Other conditions needing immediate surgery are:

Intestinal Atresia
The baby vomits and does not pass stool and develops abdominal distention, that is, the tummy becomes big.

Hirschsprung's disease
It may manifest itself in vomiting and delayed passage of meconium, that is, the dark brown or black stool passed by the baby at birth.

Some conditions are present at birth, but require planned surgery, that is, there is no need to do emergency surgery:

Umbilical Hernia
Often waiting and watching a while will allow the hernia effect to close spontaneously.

Hypospadias
The urethral opening is on the underside (ventral aspect) of the penis and the penis is curved.

Epispadias
The urethral opening is on the upper side (dorsal aspect) of the penis and the penis appears short.

Extrophy Bladder
The bladder and the urethra are open.

Hernia Hydrocele, Inguinal Hernias, Undescended Testes
These are best operated at about 2 to 3 months. Hydroceles often resolve themselves. Undescended testes, if they do not come down to the scrotum in one year, require surgical intervention.

Ambiguous Genitalia
Another problem that is perplexing is ambiguous genitalia—boy or girl? The parents are anxious and sometimes even doctors do not have an immediate answer. It is helpful to have the history of the mother: if she has had some androgenic hormones during pregnancy, or if there are other female children who have a large phallus. The latter suggests a diagnosis of congenital adrenal hyperplasia—a condition in girls who have an enlarged clitoris. Specialized X-rays help us to diagnose a male who has undescended testes and has a small phallus.

Sometimes the baby is truly intersex and with the help of hormonal and chromosomal studies we can designate and make the baby a male or a female according to circumstances. The patient should be assessed by a paediatrician and a paediatric surgeon, to discuss the further course of action.

Dr Meera Luthra
M.S., M.Ch. DNB (Paediatric Surgery)
Senior Consultant Surgeon

19 TERATOGENESIS

TERATOGENESIS MEANS THE formation of abnormalities in the baby during intra-uterine life. The factors that lead to formation of these abnormalities are known as teratogens. Such abnormalities may be obvious when the baby is born or may remain undetected for a long time after birth. The degree of such abnormalities, if present, depends upon a large number of factors—to name a few, the genetic make-up of the baby, the period of gestation (pregnancy), the maternal health at the time of exposure to the teratogen, and the intensity and duration of exposure of the mother to the teratogen.

Factors which lead to teratogenesis are as follows:

INFECTIONS

Infections in the mother, like viral infections, bacterial infections and a few fungal infections. Any micro-organisms or the toxins released by them, which cross the placenta and reach the baby, might interfere with the growth and development of the baby, thereby leading to malformation in the baby.

ADDICTIONS

Drugs, liquor, smoking and other addictions like tobacco chewing, etc., in the mother. These cross the placental barrier and might damage the baby. If the damage is too intense, it might lead to abortion. If the damage is of lesser intensity, the baby is born an addict to any of these agents.

CHEMICAL FACTORS

Long-term antibiotics, anti-psychotic drugs like anti-depressants, mood elevators, sleeping pills, etc.

Drugs used for cancer treatment and hormones given as a therapeutic measure will have teratogenic effects if the woman happens to be pregnant during such treatment. Such pregnancies might be terminated to save the life of the mother.

PHYSICAL AGENTS

- Lowering of oxygen pressure in the blood of the mother during flights. This is unlikely to happen in modern aircrafts, unless there is a fall in cabin pressure, in which case the mother-to-be should grasp the oxygen mask and breathe deeply. Also, she should avoid visits to high

altitude areas like Ladakh, for the same reason.
- Exposure to X-rays, physical violence, trauma, radiation from sources like atom bombs, solar eclipse, etc., can turn out to be harmful for both mother and baby. Physical trauma can occur from rough journeys, sports like horse riding, trekking, mountaineering, or gymnastics undertaken during sexual activities.

INDUSTRIAL POLLUTION

This is relevant for women employed in various industries. Casual exposure to pollution is not likely to have noticeable effects.

MALNUTRITION

Vitamin and mineral deficiencies can cause inadequate or underdevelopment of the baby.

It is very important for every pregnant woman to realize that she should protect herself from the above mentioned factors, which might lead to fetal abnormalities, especially if she is exposed to these factors during the first 4 months of pregnancy.

These factors might either affect the placenta or, if they cross the placental barrier and reach the baby, interfere with its growth and development.

PRECAUTIONS TO BE TAKEN DURING PREGNANCY

Relax mentally and physically, so that you do not need any medicines to keep you calm. Over-exhaustion can cause sleeplessness. Short periods of rest twice or thrice during the day are recommended.

- Eat a balanced diet. The golden rule about diet is, 'Eat a little bit of every food item but excess of nothing.' If necessary, consult your doctor for supplementation of vitamins, iron, calcium, etc. Some women get morning sickness or vomit a lot or do not feel like eating. These women should avoid foods which lead to gastric irritation and they should eat small quantities of nourishing food more frequently during the afternoons or evenings when the nausea is relatively less.
- Nowadays, young women want to maintain their slim figures. Some women think that if they eat less, their babies will be smaller and they will have an easier delivery. The fetus is like a parasite and it will draw all the nutrition it needs whether the mother has enough or not. This results in malnourishment of the mother. It is advisable that the mother eats an adequate quantity of a well-balanced diet.
- Avoid consuming liquor, tobacco or any habit-forming drugs. It is wise to avoid the company of addicts. This will keep you away from temptation and social pressures to consume such items. Spending time in the company of smokers leads to passive smoking on the part of the mother.
- Protect yourself from all kinds of infections. Do not visit sick relatives or friends. Send a bouquet of flowers or a 'get well' card instead. Avoid

visits to hospitals as you are likely to be exposed to a large number of infections. Avoid going to crowded places like cinema halls, markets, and the like.
- Protect yourself from physical agents like fatigue, exhaustion, jerky journeys, joyrides in amusement parks, horse riding, etc.
- Avoid taking medicines altogether, if you can. If you get a headache or a backache use a pain balm instead of pain killers.
- Avoid being X-rayed. Tell your doctor about your pregnancy.

Do not be over-anxious about teratogenesis; or your mental tension will create problems for you. Take time off to relax mentally and physically Remember, 50% of your baby's health depends upon hereditary factors and the other 50% depends upon how well you look after yourself.

During this period, members of your family tend to pamper you. Make the most of it and allow yourself to be looked after by them. This is their way of looking after you and your baby. If you feel that they are not giving you enough attention, then do not get into spells of depression. Instead, go out of your way and look after yourself, and the baby will be looked after automatically by you.

Dr Asha Singh
MBBS, MS, Ph.D (Genetics),
Prof. of Anatomy,
Maulana Azad Medical College, New Delhi

RECOMMENDED READING

- **Pregnancy and Birth along with Practical Tips**

The New Pregnancy & Childbirth: Choices & Challenges
Sheila Kitzinger

The Encyclopaedia of Pregnancy and Birth
Janet Balaskas, Yehudi Gordon

Active Birth
Janet Balaskas

- **A new look at birth, stressing on the calm and quiet aspects of birth**

Birth without Violence
Dr Frederick Leboyer

Birth Reborn
Dr Michel Odent

Magical Child
J.C. Pearce

This book will help you rediscover Nature's plan for our children. It also discusses childbirth.

- **Breastfeeding**

The Breastfeeding Book
Marie Messenger Davis

Helping Mothers to Breastfeed
Felicity Savage and R.K. Anand
Available from: Association for Consumer Action on Safety and Health (ACASH) P.O. Box 2498, Mumbai 400002

The Womanly Art of Breastfeeding
La Leche League International

- **Childcare**

Dr R.K. Anand's Guide to Childcare
Dr R.K. Anand

This book is also available online. If you are travelling and need to consult it when the baby falls ill, go to www.guidetochildcare.org

Baby and Childcare
Dr R.K. Suneja
This includes addresses of institutions for the handicapped, Thallassemics India Main Center for Genetic Studies

- **Parenting**

What do you really want from your children?
Dr Wayne W. Dyer

Smart Parenting
Nutan Pandit

- **Food**

Food Rules (An eater's manual)
Michael Pollan

Eating Wisely and Well
Dr Ramesh Bijlani

- **Miscellaneous**

Women's Experience of Sex
Sheila Kitzinger
A comprehensive book on sexual behaviour, feelings, difficulties, phases, grieving, etc.

Herald of Health (Magazine)
Oriental Watchman Publishing House, Post Box 1417, Salisbury Park, Pune 411037, email: owphpune@gmail.com

A family magazine for vibrant and healthy living, includes articles on latest medical updates and lifestyles.

Born To Buy
Juliet B. Schor
This book discusses the commercialized child and the new consumer culture. It will help you to become a discerning buyer.

Stop Walking On Eggshells
Paul T. Mason & Randi Kreger
Living with someone with a Borderline Personality Disorder
Do you feel manipulated, controlled or lied to?
Are you the focus of intense violent and irrational rages?
Are you 'walking on eggshells' to avoid the next confrontation?

You Can Heal Your Life
Louise L. Hay
This book will help you gain self-esteem and self-acceptance. It has a list of medical problems, the probable psychological cause of the disease and a healing affirmation you can read to heal yourself. The healing affirmations have been known to help cure many cases.

INDEX

Abdomen after delivery, 12
Abdominal examination, 17
ABIM Foundation, 102
Accidental haemorrhage, 4
Acidity, 32
ACOG American College of Obs & Gyn, 97, 102
AFP test, 14, 19
Alcohol 31, 49
Alpha-Feto-Protein test, 14
American College of Obstetricians and Gynecologists, 97, 102
American journal of Obs & Gyn, 1963, 97, 100
Amniocentesis, 14, 19
Amniotic fluid, 69
Analgesic or Anesthetic, administration of, 106-7
Anatomy, 6-9
   cervix, 7
   fallopian tubes, 7
   uterus, 6
   vagina, 6
Anemia 37
Anesthesia, 97
Antenatal check ups, 39
Antenatal visits, 13
Antibiotics, 34, 35, 97, 98, 122, 144, 146, 152, 163, 170
Antibiotic-resistance, 43
Antibodies, 37
Anti D immunoglobulin, 38, 148
Anti-Tetanus injection, 19
Antonio, Michael, 43
Apgar Score, 104
Artificial early rupture of membrane, 106
Artificial Rupture of Membranes (ARM), 86-87
Aum breathing, 62

Baby Friendly Hospital Initiative (BFHI), 105
Baby-friendly, 120
Baby's heart rate, in labour, 69
Bacillus thuringiensis (BT), 42

Backache, 41
Behavioural changes, 28-31
   abnormal cravings, 28
   alcohol, 31
   driving, 31
   medicines, 29
   mood swings, 28-29
   sleeplessness, 29
   smoking, 30
   tiredness, 28
   tobacco chewing, 30
Birth Matters, 105
Birth Reborn, 111
Birth without Violence, 110
Birth, 92-96
   baby at birth, 96
   first stage of labour, 92
   gentle contractions, 93
   prepared childbirth, 94
   risk factors, 93
   second stage of labour, 93-94
   third stage of labour, 95-96
   unnatural or difficult birth, 93
Bleeding, red, 69
Blocked ducts, 145-46
Blood banks, 97
Blood tests during Pregnancy, 13-16
   AFP-Alpha-Feto-Protein test, 14
   double marker test, 14-15
   haemoglobin levels, 13
   HIV/AIDS, 16
   Pets, Gardening, Raw Meat (Toxoplasma), 15-16
   TORCH tests, 15
   triple marker test, 14
   urine test, 10, 16
   VDRL test, 14
Body's design for birth, 3-4
Body weight, 47-48

Bourne, Gordon, 10
Boy or Girl?, 20–21
   douching, 20–21
   diet theory, 20
   potassium tablet, 20
   temperature method, 20
   timing of intercourse, 20
Brain, 2
Breast Abscess, 147
Breast pump, 127–28, 146
Breast stimulation, 67, 88
Breastfeeding, 113–51
   at birth, 119–20
   baby's nose gets blocked, 129–30
   bonding, 136–37
   bottle vs nipple, 140
   bottle-feeding, 142
   bottles sterilization, 141–42
   bra size, 118
   breast pumps, 127–28
   breast size, 116–17
   breast vs bottle, 137
   burping the baby, 134
   colostrum, 115–16, 124
   constant feeding demand, 121
   contraceptive effects of, 137
   correct sucking, 115
   correct way to feed, 114–15
   cow's milk, 141
   diet, 49
   duration of, 138–39
   engorgement, 126–27
   exclusive breastfeeding, 120–21
   express breast milk, 127
   fat-rich hind milk, 116
   feeding bras, 117–18
   feeding time, 130–31
   flat nipples, 119
   foremilk, 132
   forerunner to milk, 124
   hind milk, 132
   how to feed expressed breast milk, 129
   how to position the baby, 134–35
   immediate breastfeeding, 104–5
   important for baby, 113
   leaking breasts, 121
   less milk, 133–34
   let down reflex, 121
   mature milk, 126
   medication, 122
   milk powder, 140–41
   myths, 137–38
   night feed, 131–32
   position after caesarean birth, 135
   positioning of twins, 136
   preparation for feeding, 122–23
   problems during, 143–44
      blocked ducts, 145–46
      cleft palate, 150
      feeding a baby by cup, 150–51
      feeding in the incubator, 147
      feeding low birth weight, 147–48
      Jaundice, 148–50
      Mastitis (inflammation of the breast), 146
      premature babies, 147–48
      Thrush/Candida infection, 144–45
   rooming-in, 120
   second night syndrome, 124–25
   storing breast milk, 128–29
   twins, 136
Breathing and relaxation, 76–83
   breathing focus, 78
   breathing for labour, 77
   breathing patterns, 78–80
   chest-level breathing, 78–79
   concentration breathing, 80
   conditioned reflex, 77
   deep cleansing breath, 78
   distraction breathing, 80–81
   ignorance-fear-tension-pain syndrome, 76
   jaw-level breathing, 'out', 79–80
   not-pushing breathing, 81
   pushing breathing, 82–83
   quick relaxation in labour, 76–77
   transition breathing, 81–82
   waist-level breathing, 78
Breathing techniques, 5
Breech babies, 9, 111
Breast pump
   battery operated type, 128
   bulb type, 128
   electric type, 128
   syringe type, 128
   See also Breastfeeding
Brewer, Tom, 48
British Medical Journal, 98
BT Toxin, 42

Caesarean section, 4, 35, 57, 67, 69, 83, 85, 87, 90, 97–99, 104, 106–7, 112, 136, 155–56, 157
   bleeding/sex, 157–58
   exercises after removal of stitches, 157
   exercises after, 155
   exercises before stitches are removed, 156–57
   planned caesarean, 85
   position for breastfeeding, 135
Caffeine, 46
Calories, 39, 46, 49, 51
Carbon Monoxide, 30
Cervix, effaced, 68
Childbirth Without Fear, 4–5
Chocolates, 28, 45–47, 50–51
'Choosing Wisely', 101–2
Cleft Palate, 150
Coffee, 46
Cola drinks, 12, 46
Colostrum, 105, 115–16, 119–20, 122–26, 130, 138, 147, 149.
   See also Breastfeeding
Common Obstetric Problems, 106
Complications at birth, 7
Conditions needing special attention, 35–36
   high blood pressure, 35–36
   vaginal bleeding, 35
Conscious 'breathing', 107
Contractions, real, false, 68
Contraception, 160–67
   abstinence, 160
   billings method, 162
   breastfeeding, 162–63
   checking the cervical mucus, 162
   coitus interruptus, 160
   condom, 165
   diaphragm or the cervical cap, 165
     intra-uterine device (IUD), 164
   medicine for abortion, 166
   morning-after contraception, 165
   pills, 163–64
   rhythm method, 160–61
   spermicidal pessaries, 165
   surgical sterilization, 166
   temperature method, 161–62
   withdrawal method, 160
Cotton seed oil, 44
Cow's milk, 141. *See also* Breastfeeding
CrylAb, insecticidal protein, 43
cystitis, 34

Dais (midwives), 111
Diarrhoea, Home Remedy for, 33
Diabetes, 11–12, 16, 18, 38–39, 88–90, 93, 106, 163
   diet, 39
   gestational diabetes, 39, 90
Diastolic blood pressure, 36
Diet in Labour, 48–49
Diet theory, 20
Digestive problems, 31–33
   Constipation, 33
   diarrhoea, 33
   heartburn, 32
   nausea, 31–32
   piles, 33
   vomiting, 31–32
Dizzy, 37, 79
DNA sequence, 12
Doctor
   Dr Dick Read, 95
   Dr Lamaze, 78, 95
   Dr Michel Odent, 95, 110, 111, 112
   Dr Nirmala Kesaree, 119
   Dr Craigin, 97
   Dr Kerr, 97
   Dr Kloosterman, 98
   Dr Wagner, 106
   Dr Ian Donald, 106
   Dr R.D. Laing, 110
   Dr Fredrick Leboyer, 110, 112
Double marker test, 14–15
Down's Syndrome, 12, 15, 19
Driving, 31
Dressed to Kill, the link between breast cancer and bras, 117
Driving, 31
Drugs, analgesics and anesthetics, 93

Eclampsia, 36
Ectopic pregnancy, 7, 164, 166
Endorphin hormones, 2, 94, 111
Enema, 86, 92
Epigenetics, 12
Essential amino acids, 42
Estrogen hormone, 42
Estimated date of delivery, 84–85, 88–89, 123, 148
Exercises after a normal delivery, 154
Exercises during pregnancy, 54–64
   ankle movements, 57
   arches of the foot, 61
   aum breathing, 62

bust exercise, 55–56
curling leaf, 59
deep breathing, 55
forward backward, 58
grounding, 54
knee-chest position, 58–59
leg lift, 59
leg swing, 60
neck exercise, 54–55
pelvic floor exercise, 56–57
pelvic lift, 58
pelvic tilting, 60–61
precautions, 57
relaxation, 62–63
shoulder rotation, 55
squatting, 61–62
walking for cramps, 61
Exon skipping technique, 12
Expected weight increase, 47
Experiences of Women, 4–5

Fat deposits, 49
Fears, 1, 4–5, 64
Female pelvis, 3
FHR Fetal Heart Rate, 69
Fits, 36
Flat nipples, 119
Flatulence, 33
Fluid intake, 92
Flying, 29, 30
Foods, 40–42
    calcium, 41
    iron, 40–41
    protein, 41–42
Food pyramid, 45
Freedom and Choices in Childbirth, 106
Fried foods, 47

Genetic solutions, 12
Genetically modified crops, 42–43
   strict labelling laws, 42
Genetically modified crops in India, 44
Genetically modified Soya Crops, 42
Genetically modified Foods, 43
Genetics, 12, 43, 172
Gentle birth, 109–12
German Measles, 38
Gestational diabetes, 39, 90. *See also* Diabetes
Ghee, 47–49, 51, 123, 139

Glucose tolerance test, 90. *See also* Diabetes

Haemoglobin levels, drop, 37
Happy, being, 11
HCG, Human Chorionic Gonadotrophin hormone, 10, 14, 15, 31
Headache, 36
Healthy Foods Pyramid, 45
Hiccups, 134
Hippocratic Oath, 101
HIV or AIDS, 16
Home inductions, 88–89
   breast stimulation, 88–89
Horizontal scar, 98
Human digestive tract, 43
Hunger pangs, 52
Hyperemesis, 32
Hypertension, 12, 36, 85

Ignorance-Fear-Tension-Pain Syndrome, 76
Impairment of circulation, 2
Indian sweets, 47
Induction methods, 86–88
   artificial rupture of membranes, 86–87
   castor oil, 86
   gel or pessary, 86
   indications for intravenous drip, 88
   intramuscular injection, 87
   intravenous drip, 87–88
   sweeping and stretching, 86
Intercourse, 2, 6, 20–21, 35, 65–67, 69, 89, 158, 160, 162–63, 165–66
Internal vaginal examination, 10, 16–17, 86
Intra uterine contraceptive device, 99
Irritability, 41
IUGR, Intra Uterine Growth Restriction, 30

Jaggery 40, 42, 47
Jaundice, 148–50
   abnormal jaundice, 148
   breast milk jaundice, 149
   phototherapy, 149
   physiological jaundice, 149
Joints, xi, xii, 3, 27, 38, 51, 54, 58, 60, 61, 73
Journal Obstetrics & Gynaecology (British Commonwealth), 100

Ketones, 16, 32

Labelling laws, 42
Labour time, 68–75
    all-fours position, 72
    back massage, 74
    back to back, 75
    backache, 72
    comforters, 73–74
    effleurage, 73–74
    fluid leak, 69
    hand squeeze, 73
    in case water bag bursts, 71
    kneeling, 72
    leg massage, 74
    onset signs, 68
    palming, 73
    positions to adopt, 70
    precaution, 70
    sitting on the bed, 72–73
    standing with back to wall, 72
    upright position for labour, 71–72
    urgent medical attention, 69
    using a dining chair, 71
    walking, 71
Laing, Dr R.D., 110
Lancet, 103
Leboyer, Dr Frederick, 110

Maida, 47
Masala curry, 47
Mastitis (Inflammation of the breast), 130, 137, 144–47
    prevention of, 146
Maternal mortality, 97
Mayes' Midwifery, 18
Meals, several, 31
Medical termination of pregnancy, 19–20, 38, 164
Methods of cooking, 46
Midwives Information & Research Service, 104
Milk power, 140. *See also* Breastfeeding
Miscarriage, 13, 29, 35, 38, 91
Missed period, 10, 166
Mithai, 47
Mood swings, 28–29
Muscle action, 3, 76
Muscular dystrophy, 12

Natural childbirth, 5, 51, 102
Next Gen Sequencing, 12
Nicotine, 30
Nirmala Kesaree method, 119. *See* Flat nipples

Non-pharmacological methods, 5
Non-Stress Test (NST), 18–19
Non-vegetarians, 42
Normal birth, 152–53
    avoid spicy foods, 153
    avoidable exercises, 153
    contractions while feeding, 152
    discomfort, 152
    overstrain, 153
    pelvic floor exercises, 153
    stretch marks, 153

Obstetrics and the Newborn, 89
Odent, Dr Michel, 95, 110–11
Organic foods, 44–45
Oxytocin, 67, 74, 83, 87–88, 105–6, 123, 125

Pain
    due to ectopic pregnancy, 7
    impairment of circulation, 2
    in groin, 27
    leg cramps, 24
    perception, 1–2
    on caesarean scar, 98
    sides of abdomen, 27
    under the breasts, 27
    uterine contractions, 4
Painkillers, 2, 70, 94
Papa, Francois, 20
Pharmacological anesthesia, 104
Physical changes, 22–28
    backache, 26–27
    breast changes, 22
    darkening pigmentation, 22
    dizziness, 25
    fainting, 25
    footwear, 26
    itching, 25
    leg cramps, 24
    nasal congestion, 26
    pain in the groin and sides of abdomen, 27
    pain under the breasts, 27
    palpitations, 24–25
    shortness of breath, 24
    stretch marks, 25–26
    swollen hands and feet, 28
    teeth and gums, 23
    tingling and numbness, 27
    varicose veins, 22–23

Physicians for compassionate care, 101
Physiotherapist, 4
Pickles, 28, 44–46
Piles, 33
Placental insufficiency, 89
Planning a Healthy Baby, 11
Post-natal Depression, 158
Potatoes, 32, 39, 43, 45–46, 49–50, 52
Practical Obstetric Problems, 86
Precautions to be taken during pregnancy, 171–72
Pre-Conception Care, 12–13
Preconditioned breathing, 95
Premature babies, 94, 98, 115, 123, 125, 140, 147–48
Premature labour, 29, 36, 65, 67
Premature Rupture of Membranes (PPROM). *See also* Artificial Rupture of Membrane (ARM), 87
Primitive consciousness, 95, 110
Prolonged pregnancy, 89–91
   diabetic mother, 90
   fetal heart rate, 89
   placental insufficiency I.U.G.R., 89–90
   prolonged labour, 91
   rhesus-negative, 91
   toxaemia, 90–91
   very high blood pressure, 91
   water bag bursting, 91
Protein, 41

Read, Dick, 4–5
Relaxation techniques, 93, 107
Reproductive Toxicology, 43
Rhesus-negative blood group, 13, 37
Royal College of Midwives, 104
Royal College of Obstetricians & Gynaecologists, 104
Rubella, 38
Rupture of Membranes, 87. *See also* Artificial Rupture of Membrane (ARM)

Sacro-iliac joints, 3
Safer Childbirth?, 18
Salk, Lee, 11
Scar rupture, signs of, 9–100
Seasonal fruits & vegetables, 46
Second Night Syndrome, 124–25
Sedatives, 94
Sex during pregnancy, 65–67
   after the birth, 67
   bleeding, 66
   breast stimulation, 67
   feeling, 65
   intercourse, 66–67
   positions, 65
   precaution, 65
Sex hormones, 7, 10
Silent Knife, 99
Skin to skin, 124–26
Sleeplessness, 29
Sling for the baby, 154
Smoking, 30
Soya, 43
Soya bean, 42
Soya products, 43
Special beds, 95
Spontaneous Rupture of Membranes (SROM), 87
Sprouts, sprouted whole dal, 44
Stool of Babies, 120
Stretch marks, 22, 25–26, 60, 153
Stretch marks, 25–26
sugar substitutes, 46, 47
Surgery at Birth, conditions, requiring, 168–69
   Ambiguous Genitalia, 169
   Diaphragmatic Hernia, 168
   Epispadias, 169
   Extrophy Bladder, 169
   Gastroschisis, 168
   Hernia Hydrocele, 169
   Hirschsprung's disease, 169
   Hypospadias, 169
   Imperforate anus, 168
   Inguinal Hernias, 169
   Intestinal Atresia, 169
   Oesophageal Atresia, 168
   Omphalocoel, 168
   Tracheo-Oesophageal Fistula, 168
   Umbilical Hernia, 169
   Undescended Testes, 169
Sympathetic caring companion, 107
Sympathetic Nervous System, 2–3
Symphysis pubis, 3
Syntocin, 87. *See also* Oxytocin
Syntocinon, 69. *See also* Labour time

Taxoplasma, 15
Tea, 10, 12, 31–34, 46, 49–50, 53
Teratogenesis, 170–72
   addictions, 170
   chemical factors, 170
   factors, 170–71
   industrial pollution, 171

    infections, 170
    malnutrition, 171
    physical agents, 170–72
Tew, Marjorie, 18
Thalassaemia, 12
Thalidomide tragedy, 10
Threatened abortion, 66
Thrush/Candida infection, 144–45
Thumb sucking, 9
Tabacco, smoking, chewing, male fetus, 30
TORCH test, 15
Toxaemia, 36–39, 48, 85, 88, 90
Traditional recipes, 50
Trans-Vaginal ultrasound, 18
Trauma of birth, 109
Trauma of labour, 109
Travelling, car, train, auto, 29
Triple marker test, 14
Triplet and quadruplet pregnancies, 84
Twin pregnancy, 24, 84

Ultrasound, 12, 14–15, 17–20, 98–99, 107, 166
   measurements of the uterine scar, 99
ultrasound safety, 18
Umbilical Cord, xi, xii, 8, 9, 27, 43, 70, 95, 109-111
Urinary tract infection, 33–35, 152
    cystitis, 34
    frequent urination, 33
    urinary tract infection, 34
    vaginal discharge, 34–35
Urine Test, 16, 36

Uterine scar, layered healing of, 100
Uterine rupture, 97
Under nutrition in mother, 48

Vaginal Birth after a Caesarean Section (VBAC), 97–102
    caesarean scar or incision, 98–99
VDRL test, 14
vegetables, 49
Verma, I.C., 12
Vertical incision, 98
Vitamins, Fat soluble A, D, E and K
Vitamin D, 41
vomiting and nausea, 31, 32, 36

Weight, 46, 47, 48, 49
Water leak, coloured, 69
Weight Control, 51–53
   avoid temptation, 52
   discourage food gifts, 53
   do not diet, 53
   limit your portions, 52
   professional consultancy, 53
   regular eating, 51–52
   relax, 51
   silent efforts, 52
   water intake, 52–53
   weigh regularly, 52
Weight increase in pregnancy, 47, 48
Wholesome foods, 44–46
Williams Obstetrics, 100
World Health Organization (WHO), 102–3